Embrace Your Special Needs Child, Prayer, and Parenting

Find the Faith and Courage to Be a Great Parent for Your Child

By: Maria Cruz & Patrick Baldwin

Copyright 2018
American Christian Defense Alliance, Inc.
Baltimore, Maryland
ACDAInc.Org

All Rights Reserved. No part of this publication may be reproduced in any form or by any means, including scanning, photocopying, or otherwise without prior written permission of the copyright holder.

Embrace Your Special Needs Child, Prayer, and Parenting
Special Request

Thank you for purchasing our book and supporting our Ministry. We actually have two requests – To Pray for Our Ministry and to Read this Book All the Way through. No Ministry can Survive without Prayers and Support so we ask you to keep our Ministry in Your Daily Prayers and Pray as the Lord leads.

We encourage you to Read the Book you purchased all the way through. Many Books NEVER Get Read, and the ones that do only get read the first few pages.

One of our Special Request is that if you are serious about learning the material in this book that you take time to actually read this book in its entirety – all the way through.

We all lead such busy lives nowadays and can get side tracked so easily, please take a moment to consider my words and read to the end of the book and keep us in Your Prayers.

Thank You once again for purchase. We deeply appreciate Your Prayers and Support and know that God will Bless You as You continue to Bless this Ministry.

Embrace Your Special Needs Child, Prayer, and Parenting

Table of Contents

Special Request 2

Embracing Pregnancy, Your Child, and Parenting...................... 7

Chapter 1: Handle With Care 8

Chapter 2: The Miracle of Life 15

Chapter 3: Meant to be Parents... 20

Chapter 4: We're Having a Baby 26

Chapter 5: The First Trimester 34

Chapter 6: The Second Trimester.. 41

Chapter 7: The Third Trimester 47

Chapter 8: Let's Do This 54

Chapter 9: Family 59

Chapter 10: Children are the Future 63

Parenting Special Needs Children 66

Prelude... 67

Chapter 1: You Are Going to be the Parent of a Special Needs Child 68

Chapter 2: Guarding Your Heart, Soul, Mind, and Strength ... 75

Chapter 3: True Love is Devoid of All Pride 98

Chapter 4: Overcoming the Educational Obstacles.............. 107

Chapter 5: We Are Family 113

Chapter 6: Let Your "Light" Shine...................................... 118

Chapter 7: Dealing With Special Social and Communication Needs 124

Chapter 8: Dealing With Special Neurological Needs 129

Chapter 9: Dealing with Genetic and Physical Special Needs 135

Chapter 10: Your Not-So-Secret Secret Thoughts 144

Prayer 148

Disclaimer.. 149

Preface 151

Chapter 1: What is Prayer? 153

Chapter 2: How to Pray 166

Chapter 3: Why Pray 177

Chapter 4: Making Time to Pray.. 184

Chapter 5: Praying the Scriptures 194

Chapter 6: Praying for God's Will to be Done 202

Chapter 7: Jesus Example of Prayer 205

Chapter 8: Learning to be a Prayer Warrior............................. 225

Chapter 9: Praying for Healing... 242

Chapter 10: Praying as a Means of Spiritual Warfare 248

Chapter 11: Developing Your Prayer List 260

Chapter 12: When It Seems God Doesn't Hear Your Prayers.... 265

Chapter 13: Fasting and Prayer 268

Chapter 14: Prayer-Conclusion... 285

Special Gift 289

Stay in Contact 291

Find All Our Books 292

Additional Formats 294

Embrace Your Special Needs Child, Prayer, and Parenting

Embracing Pregnancy, Your Child, and Parenting

YOUR GUIDE BOOK TO LEARN HOW TO UNLOCK THE SECRETS OF SUCCESSFUL PARENTING

By: Maria Cruz & Patrick Baldwin

Chapter 1: Handle With Care

Psalm 127:3 says, *Children are a heritage from the Lord, offspring a reward from Him.*

…from the LORD—that's where our children come from. The LORD. He entrusts them to us to care for; helping them go from infancy to adulthood safely, securely, and in an atmosphere that reflects God's love as much as is humanly possible.

There are a number of verses and passages of scripture in the Bible that reflect and teach this truth. We'll be looking at several of them throughout the pages of this book. I want to begin, however, by taking a look into the heart and mind of the woman I consider to be the most Godly mother of all times. Her name: Hannah.

We are introduced to Hannah in the first chapter of the Old Testament book of First Samuel. Hannah, who is one of Elkanah's two wives, is a tender-hearted and Godly woman who desperately longs to be a mother.

Her inability to conceive a child is something Peninnah, Elkanah's other wife, takes great pleasure in. Peninnah's taunting and ridicule plants seeds of insecurity and doubt in Hannah's mind; doubts that Elkanah quickly puts to rest; assuring his sweet wife that his love for her is true—child or no child.

I'm sure this had to bring at least some degree of comfort to Hannah's heart and mind, but it didn't change the fact that Hannah wanted to be a mom more than anything in the world. Hannah knew, though, that wanting to be a mom wasn't enough. Hannah knew that the gift of motherhood came from one 'place' and one 'place' only—God.

So Hannah prayed. She prayed and she prayed and she prayed some more. But her prayers weren't 'just' to become a mom. Hannah told God that if He would bless her with a child she would give the child back to him—literally. She told God that if He would bless her with a son she would give him to Eli to be raised up as the next High Priest and Judge over all of Israel.

After praying the prayer Hannah and Elkanah conceived a child. When the baby was born they named him Samuel. And true to her word, when Samuel was about three or four years old Hannah took him to live in the Tabernacle with Eli so that he could learn the duties of the priesthood. Samuel grew up to be a man of deep faith and one who obeyed God to the letter. He was the last Judge of Israel before they demanded that He appoint someone to be their king.

I'm sharing Hannah's story with you to remind you that your children are on loan to you from God. You are their caretakers and their role models. God has charged you with the task, aka, given you the privilege of overseeing some of His most priceless treasures.

As a steward of these treasures you need to be sure you care for them the way God expects you to—the way He told us to in Deuteronomy 6:5-9:

And thou shalt love the Lord thy God with all thine heart, and with all thy soul, and with all thy might. And these words, which I command thee this day, shall be in thine heart: And thou shalt teach them diligently unto thy children, and shalt talk of them when thou sittest in thine house, and when thou walkest by the way, and when thou liest down, and when thou risest up. And thou shalt bind them for a sign upon thine hand, and they shall be as frontlets between thine eyes. And thou shalt write them upon the posts of thy house, and on thy gates.

You are to teach them diligently. When you teach diligently you teach consistently; meaning on a regular basis. But teaching with diligence also implies that you are meticulous and careful to make sure they don't just know *about* God, but that they know who God *is*—His character.

God doesn't just tell us the manner in which we are supposed to teach our children. No, God also gives us the specifics of how to get the job done. He tells us to **talk of them when thou sittest in thine house, and when thou walkest by the way.** He goes on to say we are to teach our children when they lay down and when they are awake. In other words, the Word of God is to permeate our children's lives. Their exposure to God's Word needs to be the norm—not the exception. We are to **teach our children to see God** in everything, **give thanks** to God for all things, **give God the credit** He is due, and **give God total control** of our lives.

And then He gets to the really personal part. Teaching our children these things needs to be done by example. Children really do learn what they live, and God is calling us to make sure they live in homes where God is first and foremost every day and in every way.

That's a pretty tall order—an awesome responsibility. It is not impossible, though, because God never gives you a job to do without also providing you with the resources necessary to do it…and do it well.

The Word of God …prayer…the Holy Spirit…Godly counsel from other parents…a parent-heart that wants to give their children the best life possible—these are the resources we have at our disposal.

You need to know, however, that these resources aren't meant to be optional. Deuteronomy 6 isn't a suggestion or a wish. It is a command from the creator to the moms and dads He entrusts with His most priceless treasures.

Hannah knew she was raising Samuel *for* God. Raising your children *for* God is your job, too.

Chapter 2: The Miracle of Life

Have you ever looked at a newborn baby? I mean really looked—their tiny fingernails, the perfect little curvatures of their ears, the soft little eyelashes, the way they instinctively know when Mom is nearby? They are pure perfection, aren't they? They are also a living, breathing miracle.

Yes, life is a miracle. It couldn't just happen by accident. Too many things have to be just right in order for an egg and sperm to get together and stay that way. Oh, I know there are those first-time-I-had-sex-I-got-pregnant people out there. But they are far from the norm. In fact, the UK's Daily Mail website and the New York Post newspaper reported that research conducted on three thousand couples showed that on average, it takes couples one hundred and four sessions of lovemaking before pregnancy is achieved.

Additional research shows that less than half of all couples get pregnant within the first six months of trying to conceive, but that just over ninety percent conceive within a year. So like I said, there's nothing accidental or coincidental about it.

I also know that getting the news that you are expecting can take you on a rollercoaster of emotions. Excitement, disbelief, anxiousness, fear, awe, surprise, elation…and sometimes disappointment and anger are the most common.

Not every pregnancy is planned or desired. Most teenagers aren't trying to achieve pregnancy when they're in the back seat of a car or home alone on the couch. Sometimes couples don't feel ready to start a family for one reason or another, but find out they are anyway. Other couples feel their families are complete and/or are getting ready to be empty-nesters when suddenly….

For others—especially couples who have experienced the grief of miscarriage or infertility—pregnancies can be scary. They want it so badly they are too afraid to let themselves enjoy it. They don't want to get their hopes up only to have their hearts broken again.

And then there are those that count down the days from the time their chances of conceiving were the highest until they can take a pregnancy test to see if this will be the month.

No matter what you are feeling or thinking, though, you need to know that God knows exactly what's going on and he knows exactly what He is doing. He knew wayyyyyyyyy back when he said, "Let there be light…" when each of us would be conceived. I know that's a lot to wrap your head around, but it's true. The Bible says so in Psalm 139:15-16:

My frame was not hidden from You, When I was made in secret, And skillfully wrought in the lowest parts of the earth. Your eyes saw my substance, being yet unformed. And in Your book they all were written, The days fashioned for me, When as yet there were none of them. (NKJV)

Every mother out there can testify that giving birth and being a parent is truly a gift from God – The Miracle of Life if you would. Hopefully God will see fit in His plan to bless you abundantly with children in the near future. Just remember Children have angels assigned to watch over them so make sure you're gracious to strangers.

Hebrews 13:2 says, "Do not forget to show hospitality to strangers, for by so doing some people have shown hospitality to angels without knowing it."

As far as I know I've never welcomed an actual angel into my home, but I have been the recipient of their God-given ability to intervene in my life in a way that still leaves me 'on my knees thankful'.

Remember: Babies aren't made by accident. A mommy and daddy's perfect timing doesn't even guarantee anything. It is God's perfect timing that results in the miracle of life.

Chapter 3: Meant to be Parents

Genesis 1:27-28 says, *"So God created man in His own image; in the image of God He created him; male and female He created them. Then God blessed them, and God said to them, "Be fruitful and multiply; fill the earth and subdue it; have dominion over the fish of the sea, over the birds of the air, and over every living thing that moves on the earth."thing that moveth upon the earth."*

Genesis 9:1 says, *"So God blessed Noah and his sons, and said to them: "Be fruitful and multiply, and fill the earth."*

In Genesis 28:3, Isaac said to Jacob, *"May God Almighty bless you, And make you fruitful and multiply you, That you may be an assembly of peoples;*

And finally, Psalm 127:3-5 tells us, *"Lo, children are an heritage of the Lord: and the fruit of the womb is his reward. As arrows are in the hand of a mighty man; so are children of the youth. Happy is the man that hath his quiver full of them: they shall not be ashamed, but they shall speak with the enemies in the gate."*

It isn't difficult to see the common thread running through these four verses, is it?

God wants us to be parents. Next to worshipping Him and sharing the message of the Gospel to anyone and everyone we possibly can, being a parent is the most important job God gives us to do. Remember: the job of parent is synonymous with being the caretaker of God's most precious and priceless treasures...children.

Unfortunately, not every parent knows just how important their job is. If they did, the National Children's Alliance wouldn't have to report that over 700,000 children in the US are treated or receive some type of service because of abuse or neglect each and every year. Additionally, over 3 million children in this country are the subject of an intervention or protection order.

Why do you think this is? Why would anyone want to harm an innocent child? The answers to that question are varied. Some would say it is because the parents were abused or neglected, so they don't know any better. Others would say it is because these parents is not mature enough to be a parents. And still others would say that an abusive parent's actions are beyond their control because of an addiction or emotional/mental disorder. While these things may or may not be true, the real reason child abuse/neglect happen is because God is not present in the home. When God is absent from a home a lot of other things are absent, as well. Things like patience, gentleness, genuine selflessness, diligent teaching about God, and unconditional love.

As Christians we need to be conscientious about making sure God is present in our homes. We have the same perspective on parenting that God designed us to have. We need to make sure we embrace our role as parents; viewing it as a praiseworthy responsibility rather than a chore. It is a praiseworthy responsibility we need to take to heart.

Some would ask then, if being a parent is something God desires us to do, then why are there Christian couples suffering from infertility? And if being fruitful and multiplying is so important, then where does that leave couples who don't want children or those who don't marry? Are they living outside of God's will for mankind?

Infertility is an emotionally and physically painful condition. But know this...infertility is NOT a sin and it is NOT God's way of punishing someone. Infertility is a medical condition caused by a number of different things.

What's more, infertility doesn't mean you cannot be a parent. Adoption is always as possibility. The process isn't always easy and (take it from someone who knows) it is considerably more labor-intensive than having a biological child. And don't let anyone ever tell you that adoptive parents aren't parents in every sense of the word, because they are.

Choosing to be childless is not a sin, either. Christian couples choose to remain childless in order to be able to pursue their ministries without the distractions of family. Frank and Ella are an example of this mindset.

Frank and Ella spent thirty years as dedicated youth directors. Neither felt comfortable or working with small children or babies. Tweens and teens, however, were a different story. They poured themselves into ministering to young people this age and their efforts were highly effective.

So rather than having biological children of their own, this couple chose to 'have' dozens of children over the years; loving, teaching, and mentoring them to know and love the LORD. Other couples may choose not to have children for any number of reasons that are personal in nature; reasons that are between them and the LORD. For anyone to pass judgement on these people would be very wrong.

According to scripture God prefers we have children. Children are proof of the love between a man and a woman. Children are the hope of the future—both the future of this world and of the Church. So be fruitful and multiply; raising your children to know the LORD and that they are fearfully and wonderfully made by Him and for Him.

Embrace Your Special Needs Child, Prayer, and Parenting
Chapter 4: We're Having a Baby

You've been anxiously waiting for the days and weeks to pass so that you could take a pregnancy test. The day came, you took the test, and you are on 'cloud nine' because the test came back positive. YOU ARE GOING TO HAVE A BABY!

In the days immediately following, you and your spouse shared the good news with family and close friends. You've pinched yourself (literally or figuratively speaking) a few times to remind yourself you aren't dreaming—that this is actually happening. You and your spouse have already started tossing a few names around and you have already had your first mini-panic-attack over whether or not you can go through the labor process and then actually be responsible for a helpless baby. If so, relax. All of these thoughts (and a whole lot more we're getting ready to talk about) are completely normal.

They are just part of the whole pregnancy experience. Your thoughts and worries are no different than those of any other parent-to-be, so we're going to spend the next few minutes talking about the most common thoughts and concerns of parents during those first few days and weeks following the moment you find out that you are going to have a baby.

Telling your spouse

It wasn't all that long ago women didn't have the capability to find out whether or not they were pregnant until they were at least eight weeks into the pregnancy or without going to the doctor to have blood drawn to test to see if the level of the hormone, hCG is high; indicating there is a pregnancy.

It also wasn't all that long ago expectant fathers weren't nearly as involved in the pregnancy experience or the birth of their baby as most expectant fathers are today.

Expectant fathers were usually unaware pregnancy was even a possibility until their wife shares the good news.

Today things are a lot quicker, easier, and a lot more of a joint effort. The prospective parents communicate a lot more directly about the possibility of whether or not pregnancy is possible. If, however, you are an expectant mom who wants to surprise your husband with the wonderful news, there are a number of fun ways to do so.

Give your husband a baby onesie with the logo of his favorite sports team, and a note that says 'from' your baby saying can't wait to meet you Dad, a giant cookie with your approximate due-date written in icing, or a devotional book for dads - nice.

Telling your family and close friends

Your parents, grandparents, and siblings should hear the news before the general public does.

A phone call or face-to-face visit to share your good news may be a bit 'plain', but it gets the job done. If you want to spice it up a bit try gifting grandparents with a t-shirt or mug with a grandparent saying on it is always fun. Phone calls, emails, or posts on your social media are effective and sufficient for telling friends and extended family members about your pregnancy.

Telling your employer

A close friend of mine had to go to her new boss the second day she was on the job and tell him she was pregnant. The pregnancy was something she and her husband had all but given up on happening, so learning she was going to be a mother again was an answered prayer. But it was also nerve racking. She didn't know her new employer so she had no idea how he would take the news. Thankfully he was gracious and understanding and did not treat her any differently than he did any other employee.

Telling your employer should be a priority. They need to know so that you can discuss how things like prenatal appointments and maternity leave are handled. You also need to talk to the HR person to find out what your insurance does and does not cover—what your options are regarding participating providers.

While there are some jobs that might require you to go to a limited duty status or make some special arrangements for bouts of morning sickness, being on your feet too long, or other such things. You need to remember that being pregnant is not a disease or a disability. Don't treat it as such by taking advantage of your coworkers or employer.

Choosing an OBGYN

More than likely you already have a doctor who will care for you throughout your pregnancy and who will deliver your baby. You have probably been seeing them for your yearly exams.

But there are instances in which this is not the case. If for example you have to move for a job just prior to giving birth – you will need to find a new doctor.

The whole doctor situation can be a bit unnerving. You want someone you can trust, right? Someone you feel comfortable with. Because this isn't always possible it is just one more reason for you to put your faith in the Great Physician—Jesus. He is always on-call. He will never be too busy to care for you. He knows your every need and those of your baby. He is the one you can always put your trust in and know He's got your back.

Early good prenatal care is essential

No matter who your doctor is or how and when you tell everyone else about the baby growing inside of you, the most important thing you can do for yourself and your baby is to take great care of yourself physically and emotionally.

Thankfully, most expectant moms don't have any trouble tweaking their normal lifestyle or routines once they find out they are expecting. You know—things like giving up caffeine, bouncing over rough and rocky trails on an ATV, or even putting their hobby of refinishing antique furniture on hold.

I'm here to suggest, however, that you start these things before you know you are pregnant. If you are trying to get pregnant you want to create the most welcoming, healthy, and conducive environment for your growing baby as possible.

So if you are reading this book in anticipation of the day you find out you are pregnant, start making those changes today. If you are newly-pregnant there is no question that the things I mentioned above (along with several others) are no-no's for pregnant women wanting a healthy pregnancy and healthy baby.

But if there are somethings you are in question about, don't hesitate to ask your doctor.

Congratulations! This is a wonderful, special, and amazing time in your life. Enjoy it. Make it among the happiest months of your life.

Chapter 5: The First Trimester

This book combines the biological and physiological aspects of pregnancy with the spiritual aspects of pregnancy. So in addition to learning or being reminded of what is taking place inside you (or your wife) I am also going to provide you with Scriptures of encouragement and reminders that your baby is a treasure in God's storehouse of treasures, and in spite of all that He created, He sees each and every single one of us as priceless...
irreplaceable...one-of-a-kind.

Fertilization

"Do you know the time when the wild mountain goats bear young? Or can you mark when the deer gives birth? Can you number the months that they fulfill? Or do you know the time when they bear young? ~Job 39:1-2

In spite of the fact that you may be planning to try to become pregnant by charting your ovulation times, the fact remains that there is only One who knows the moment fertilization takes place and a new life begins. That One is God.

Within those first few hours when the egg and sperm join together, a new life is formed that contains chromosomes from each parent. These chromosomes determine the sex of the baby along with a host of other things – but those things I'm sure you may already know about so let's move on . . .

The earliest stages of formation

For You formed my inward parts; You covered me in my mother's womb.
~Psalm 139:13

Looking at a picture of a three week-old baby may not provide a very clear picture of what is going on inside, but wonderful things are happening.

By the end of the third week after conception, your baby's body is basically three layers of cells that are working hard to form various intricate parts of the body. The first layer of cells forms the skin, the body's nervous system, and their eyes and ears. The second layer is what grows to become the baby's heart (along with the rest of the circulatory system), their bones, muscles, and ligaments, their kidneys, and their reproductive system. The inner-most layer of cells forms the respiratory and digestive organs and systems.

A brain, spine, arms, and legs

I will praise You, for I am fearfully and wonderfully made, Marvelous are Your works, And that my soul knows very well. ~Psalm 139:14

Four weeks after your baby has been conceived, which is usually around the time most women find out they are pregnant, they are starting to develop a brain, the spinal column is forming, and arms and legs look like little buds ready to sprout to be fully infant-sized.

Your baby is growing and developing their most important parts for living a healthy, well-rounded life. This is just another reason you need to make sure you are taking proper care of yourself so that your baby receives the best of care, too.

Accepting the Child God Gives You

For the body is not one member, but many. If the foot shall say, because I am not the hand, I am not of the body; is it therefore not of the body? And if the ear shall say, Because I am not the eye, I am not of the body; is it therefore not of the body? If the whole body were an eye, where were the hearing? If the whole were hearing, where were the smelling? But now hath God set the members every one of them in the body, as it hath pleased him. ~1 Corinthians 12:14-18

Weeks five and six following conception are busy ones, to say the least. The shape of the head becomes more distinctive, as do the eyes, ears, and nose. While your baby cannot yet see, the retinas are forming; meaning and it won't be long before they can.

Fingers begin to form on the little short arms that are still yet to grow to their full length. The upper lip is formed, and the neck becomes straighter and more distinguishable.

Most amazingly of all (in my opinion, anyway) is the fact that all of this is happening to a little person about the size of a penny!

During the final weeks of the first trimester your baby's size goes from that of a penny to about the size of a credit card. By the time the first trimester comes to an end your baby also has toes, elbows, definite eyelids, buds inside the mouth that will eventually become baby teeth, red blood cells are being produced by the liver (yes, that's there, too), and their genitalia begins to make its presence known on the outside of the body.

No wonder you don't feel like your normal self

Now if God so clothes the grass of the field, which today is, and tomorrow is thrown into the oven, will He not much more clothe you, O you of little faith? "Therefore do not worry, saying, 'What shall we eat?' or 'What shall we drink?' or 'What shall we wear?' For after all these things the Gentiles seek. For your heavenly Father knows that you need all these things.. ~Matthew 6:30-32

Now that you've been given a very brief and basic rundown of what is going on inside a woman's body during those first weeks of pregnancy, do you even have to ask why they don't feel like themselves? Is it any wonder that extreme fatigue is completely normal for expectant mothers, as is nausea, aka morning sickness?

These first weeks and months can be physically and emotionally exhausting. There's no doubt about that. But as a Christian you have the promise that God can and will sustain you through this time so that you can enjoy the blessings of being a steward of one of His treasures.

Chapter 6: The Second Trimester

As you enter into the second trimester of your pregnancy, you usually begin to feel better (no more morning sickness) and your energy level begins to rise. For many women, the second trimester of pregnancy is a time when they feel better than they've ever felt. They are excited about the baby's upcoming arrival. They are enjoying the fact that they are growing a baby-bump; bringing with it all sorts of positive attention and well-wishes. Thinking about names, nursery décor, and all the other fun things that go with becoming parents seem to start taking root during the second trimester.

While everything going on, on the outside is great, what's happening on the inside is even more thrilling. Let's take a look...

Diapers not needed...yet

As you do not know what is the way of the wind, Or how the bones grow in the womb of her who is with child, So you do not know the works of God who makes everything..
~Ecclesiastes 11:5

Beginning around the eleventh week after conception (which is technically the thirteenth week of pregnancy because the two weeks between ovulation and what would have been your next period are counted) your baby begins to pee. Their pee becomes part of the amniotic fluid your baby will live in until they makes their grand appearance into the world.

Along with that major developmental milestone, your baby's bones are hardening, more red blood cells are forming in other organs, and their sex organs are becoming more distinctive.

Something new almost every day

Before I formed thee in the belly I knew thee; and before thou camest forth out of the womb I sanctified thee, and I ordained thee a prophet unto the nations. ~Jeremiah 1:5

As you progress further into your second trimester your baby starts developing more and more of the functions and characteristics they will need to live outside the womb. They develop the ability to hear, blink their eyes, and their heart is pumping around one hundred pints of blood each day. Your baby is also rolling and flipping around quite a bit, but is still too small for you to feel these movements. Don't worry, it won't be long before you do. Additionally, their digestive system is now working and they are almost as long as a dollar bill.

Reaching the halfway mark

But the very hairs of your head are all numbered. ~Matthew 10:30

During the second trimester you will hit the half-way mark of your pregnancy. It is about this time that an ultrasound can reveal to you the sex of your child (if you want to know).

Being able to recognize your baby as either a boy or a girl isn't the only significant milestone in your baby's development during this time though. Throughout the remaining weeks of the second trimester of your pregnancy you will begin to feel your baby's movements. This is one of the most exciting aspects of pregnancy. To be able to feel your baby moving around inside your body is…is…well, there really are no adequate words to fully capture the specialness of how this feels (physically or emotionally).

It is also possible for the baby's father, grandparents, or whoever else you invite, to feel the baby's movements by placing your hand on your tummy during the baby's more active times. This, too, is a very special event and a precious bonding experience for husbands and wives and for soon-to-be-dads and their unborn child.

Discovering the sex of your baby and being able to feel their movements isn't the only things that happen during these final weeks of the second trimester. There are also many significant things going on inside your baby's body.

The sound of your voice

My son, hear the instruction of thy father, and forsake not the law of thy mother: For they shall be an ornament of grace unto thy head, and chains about thy neck .~Proverbs 1:8-9

Your baby has definite times of being asleep and awake. They can even be awakened by your movements and noises outside the womb. I find this incredible, don't you!

Your baby's body is covered in the cheesy coating and a fine layer of fuzz or hair. These things both serve to keep your baby's skin from being chapped by the amniotic fluid.

Your baby's fingerprints and footprints are engraved onto their little bodies. Each one, we know, different from anyone else's every born.

Your baby can suck their thumb and recognize Mom's voice. Yes, that's right—*they know your voice before they ever see your face!*

By the end of the second trimester your baby's lungs are developing at a rapid pace; preparing them to make their grand entrance in a few months. But because the baby's lungs and their ability to suck properly are not yet fully established, it is important that you take care to keep your baby from making their entrance too soon to avoid complications. If that happens, however, just remember God is the One in Control and He has a plan for everyone including your baby.

By the time you come to the end of your second trimester your baby weighs approximately two pounds and is approximately nine inches long – and that to me is just Awesome to think about.

Chapter 7: The Third Trimester

You're almost there—'there' being the end of your pregnancy. At this point you are feeling both excited and nervous. You are getting tired of wearing maternity clothes, yet are 'certain' you'll never be able to wear anything a 'normal' woman wears again. You have days you feel energized and ready to take on the world, but then others you feel like a beached whale that can barely get one foot in front of the other. It's that whole rollercoaster effect kicking into high gear again.

This is also the point in your pregnancy when you begin getting serious about preparing the nursery, enjoy putting all those tiny little clothes in the closet and dresser drawers, and preparing for maternity leave from your job.

At this point you also need to be finalizing arrangements for childcare once you return to work—if you plan to do so. I cannot stress how important this is, because the weeks you are home with your baby after he or she arrives fly by all too quickly. In other words, you aren't going to have the time or desire to deal with this issue while on maternity leave, so it is essential you do so now.

I also want to tell you how important it is to *enjoy* these last few weeks of your pregnancy. These are special weeks in your life—weeks that cannot be replicated no matter how many children you have. Each pregnancy story is different and needs to be experienced as the miracle it truly is.

Getting ready, but not quite set to go

For we are his workmanship, created in Christ Jesus unto good works, which God hath before ordained that we should walk in them. ~Ephesians 2:10

The third and final trimester of your pregnancy is your baby's time to develop and grow into all those finishing touches that make us capable of living outside the womb. During these last few weeks your baby's hair comes in on their heads or not(it just depends on your family).

Your baby is also stretching and kicking—sometimes causing you a good deal of discomfort. For example, one mom delivered her second daughter with an extremely bruised tailbone—bruised from the inside due to the baby's near-constant kicking and jabbing –ouch! And then there are those more comical incidents surrounding the baby's movement during the last trimester. More than one expectant mom I know has had a bowl of popcorn or other snack resting on her belly, only to have it knocked off by the baby's movements.

Your baby can and will likely have hiccups; something you can feel them doing, but cannot help them with.

At the onset of the third trimester your baby will also start working quite diligently to put on weight. The added weight and layers of fat they form fill out their skin making it less wrinkled and protects their hardening bones. This protection is necessary, because even though their bones are hardening, they are still quite soft in comparison to what they will be later on. Remember—they have to be pliable enough to make it through the birth canal.

The Father's finishing touches

The spirit of God hath made me, and the breath of the Almighty hath given me life. ~Job 33:4

Thirty weeks after conception (week thirty-two of your 'official' pregnancy) your baby starts breathing practice. They are gearing up for the outside world. To this point they have breathed in and out, but it has been more instinctive than purposeful.

At this point in time the bulk of the fuzz that has covered your baby's body also begins to fall off. The degree to which this happens varies greatly in each child. As you may already know, some babies are more hairy than others when they are born. Premature babies are especially so, if born before this stage of development. The amount of baby fuzz isn't an indicator of anything being wrong with the baby. It is simply just one aspect of their unique nature showing through.

In the final weeks of gestation your baby develops the ability to detect light. They gain about an ounce of weight per day, the added weight and fat content causes their little bodies to fill out even more, and they begin positioning themselves into the birth canal.

Your doctor will likely be checking you weekly at this point to make sure everything is going as it should.

Some doctors even do an ultrasound toward the end of the pregnancy to check to make sure the umbilical cord isn't wrapped around the baby's neck, to make sure the baby's head is not so large that they feel it would be unsafe for the mother to have a vaginal delivery, and a number of other things.

It is also at this point that mothers who are having a c-section will schedule their baby's delivery. Most c-sections are scheduled to take place the week of the due date or possibly a few days prior to the due date the mother was given. This is done in an effort to avoid the baby trying to come on its own, which in most cases of mothers having C-sections, would not be a good thing.

Most C-sections are done for the sake of either the mother or child's physical condition. However, if at all possible I strongly recommend having a vaginal birth as there are many added health benefits for the baby.

Remember, the last stages of your baby's development are important to you and to them. So continue to take care of yourself and to give your baby every possible opportunity to grow and develop the way God intended them too.

Your third trimester (and pregnancy) is almost over. D-day is fast approaching.

Chapter 8: Let's Do This

At this point in your pregnancy you probably have the crib set up, you've been to childbirth classes (if you chose to take them), you have your bag packed for the hospital, and a solid birthing plan in place. You know exactly how you want things to go and you have every intention of making the birth of your child an absolutely, positively, perfectly wonderful experience.

The only thing you aren't counting on is the fact that more often than not, the best laid birthing plans fly right out the window about the time the contractions start coming around five minutes apart.

This really hurts

To the woman He said: "I will greatly multiply your sorrow and your conception; In pain you shall bring forth children; Your desire shall be for your husband, And he shall rule over you." ~Genesis 3:16

With the first baby you 'know' it's going to hurt. You've talked to other moms. You've read a few books and watched a few movies. But geez, how hard can it really be? If it was *that* bad there wouldn't be as many babies as there are. If it was *that* bad, not even sex would make it worth the 'risk'.

The thing to remember is that every women is different and every birth is different. When my wife started getting contractions I thought it was false labor and went back to sleep because I had exams the following day. However, shortly thereafter she came back in, woke me up, and said "Its Time to Go". We contacted the OBGYN and got everything we needed and headed out.

When she got to the hospital she was close to 5cm dilated. My wife no doubt is a solider and not every women could handle that as if it was no big deal but there are some.

Keep in mind my wife is just over 5' tall and weighs a little over 100lbs (not including the pregnancy weight). So if she can do it you probably can too. Just don't have any preconceived ideas about how much pain it will be because you truly don't know.

The experience of giving birth is not something you can plan for right down to your baby's first cry. There are too many variables you have no control over. Things like: where you are when your labor starts, how long the labor and delivery will take, how cooperative your baby is, how well you work with your body's natural instincts to get the job done, and the overall type of labor experience you have.

If you are reading this and think that because you are about to give birth to baby number two, don't get too smug. Every birth is different. Don't believe me? Ask any mom who has more than one child.

That thing they say about the pain being worth it…they're right

A woman, when she is in labor, has sorrow because her hour has come; but as soon as she has given birth to the child, she no longer remembers the anguish, for joy that a human being has been born into the world. ~John 16:21

I'm not going to spend a lot of time talking about the actual labor and delivery process or about the things that take place within the first few hours and days following your child's birth. Your doctor will cover all of that, and that's as it should be.

What I do want to say is that becoming a parent truly is a cause for joy and celebration. It really is the most amazing and most important thing you will ever do in this world—second only to giving your life to Christ.

So will you really forget the pain? Will the memory really go away?

The Word of God is true in all ways—including this. Though you will remember that it hurts and your memories of the event will always be there, the memories will be such that you will see the marvelous good that came from it—not the anguish and suffering you felt.

Chapter 9: Family

Welcoming a new baby into your family is news parents don't hesitate to share while having a big smile plastered across their face and heart. Think about it...how many birth announcements have you gotten that say something like, "We're as happy as we can be to announce we are now a family of three!" or "Our family is growing day by day now that baby number three has come to stay."?

Parents, grandparents, aunts, uncles, cousins should all be a part of your child's life for so many reasons. There are far too many to cover them all adequately, lets take a few minutes to cover the most important ones now...

Family provides a sense of belonging

God set up the institution of family because He knows we thrive best when we have the communion of relationships. He knows we need to be needed and need to be wanted. He knows family units and provides the sense of belonging He created us to want and need.

Family brings a sense of responsibility

Having a child changes you—or at least it should. Having a child causes you to be less selfish and more selfless. You suddenly find yourself completely and utterly responsible for another human life. You realize that what you do and how you do it affects someone else. You realize that where you go, how you act, what you say, and everything else about your life isn't just about you—it's about you and your baby.

Family becomes more important

How many new parents have you heard say something to the effect that when their baby was born their own parents (the baby's grandparents) suddenly became wiser and smarter than they'd ever been before?

News flash! The grandparents didn't suddenly become anything (other than grandparents). The wisdom and knowledge was there before the baby was born. But when faced with the awesome and daunting task of actually being a parent themselves, well….

The role of grandparent, aunt or uncle can be a precious resource in the lives of children and their parents. For a child, these extended family members can be sounding boards, people who have time when parents don't, an added source of encouragement and unconditional love, someone to teach them skills their parents don't have, someone to just hang out with, someone to whom they can give back all of these things, and someone they can look up to as an example of faith.

Those of you who have families that can bring these things into your child's life should be thankful for the blessing of family. It is something you should not take for granted and should not deprive your child of.

Those of you who do not have family to lean on and glean from, do not have to miss out completely. You can 'adopt' a family in your church. There are undoubtedly people as hungry for a family as you are.

Family isn't always about blood and DNA. It's about exhibiting the kind of love that says "I love you just because". Never forget those that claim the name of Jesus Christ and claim His Blood are Adopted into the Family of God – So You are NEVER Alone!.

Chapter 10: Children are the Future

Babies and children just add that something extra into a family's dynamics. They bring a sense of innocence, wonder, fun, and youthfulness into a home. Children also give us purpose—or at least they should. Being a parent should make you stand a little taller on the 'ladder' of integrity. They should make you think on your words before you speak them; making sure they are honest, kind, and fair. Children should make you walk a straighter path; working hard, spending your money wisely, being honest and forthright, and setting a solid example of how to live. Children should make you desire to know God more fully and to teach them to know God on a personal level, too, because children are the future of society and of the Church.

One of the most heart-rending statements I've ever heard went something like this: The worst possible feeling a parent could have is the feeling that they might not spend eternity with their children in heaven.

Ouch! That cuts deep, doesn't it? As parents we need to be mindful of the fact that we are responsible for raising our children to know the LORD and to have a desire to seek his purpose for their lives.

That being said, you need to remember that your purpose is to raise them to know these things—not live their lives for them.

We have this Promise from God . . . .

Train up a child in the way he should go, And when he is old he will not depart from it. ~Proverbs 22:6

While none of us are perfect; meaning we all make parenting mistakes (and plenty of them), if we do our job to raise our children as directed by God in the Bible, we have nothing to worry about. You can do it as God fearing Parents that seek the Living God and honor Him by following the Word of God on how to raise your children.

Don't let things discourage or frighten you, along the way. There will always be ups and downs in life but in all things God is an ever present help in a time of need – Trust in Him, Allow His Word to inspire you to become a great parent who raises awesome kids.

Do as we are told in Lamentations 2:19…

Arise, cry out in the night: in the beginning of the watches pour out thine heart like water before the face of the Lord: lift up thy hands toward him for the life of thy young children that faint for hunger in the top of every street.

In reading this book you have either learned or have been reminded of the fact that being a parent isn't just something physical that you do. Being a parent is also a spiritual act— one that God intends to be a spiritual act of worship aimed at Him.

God knows that when we see our children as the priceless treasures they are we will love, nurture, and cherish them in such a way that glorifies God.

Embrace Your Special Needs Child, Prayer, and Parenting

Parenting Special Needs Children

A Christian Guide to Parenting Children with ADHD, Autism, Asperger's, and other Psychological, Behavioral, or Physiological Disorders

By: Patrick Baldwin

Embrace Your Special Needs Child, Prayer, and Parenting

Prelude

Having worked for close to 20 years with those in our society that are considered some of the most vulnerable, I wanted to write this book to offer Biblical Guidance for the Christian Parent.

Often times we may become overwhelmed with the thoughts, responsibilities, and day to day grind that having a special needs child can bring to your life. It is critical to see Your Child through the Eyes of God and to Keep Your Focus on Jesus Christ along the Way.

I truly Pray that this book will be a Blessing to You and Your Family and hope that You will share it with other Christian Parents who may be also dealing with the challenges of Parenting a Special Needs Child.

God Bless You

Chapter 1: You Are Going to be the Parent of a Special Needs Child

When we see the little line on the pregnancy test saying there is a baby growing inside of you, the last thing you probably think about (or one of the last things) is whether or not your baby will have special needs when it comes to their physical, mental, or emotional wellbeing.

You aren't thinking about whether or not you will be able to afford special equipment they might need to live. You aren't thinking about what your insurance will and won't cover and what kind of help you can get to make up the difference. You aren't thinking about whether or not your house will 'work' for a wheelchair, if your boss will allow you to work from home or how you will juggle work and five or six doctor's appointments a month (or possibly in a week).

You aren't thinking about the fact that your baby—the one you've just 'met'—is one of the millions of children in this country that will receive some form of special education when he or she goes to school. And that's providing he or she can go to school.

No, you aren't thinking about those things at all. You are thinking about whether the baby is a boy or girl, when the due date will be, who to share the happy news with first (other than your spouse, of course), and you even start rolling possible names around in your mind. In other words, your thoughts are focused on the joy that comes from bringing a new baby into this world.

Well guess what? Bringing a new baby into this world regardless of whether or not they have special needs *is* a joy. Each and every tiny little life that takes their first breath after working their way into this world is a cause for celebration and joy *because* we are all fearfully and wonderfully made by the LORD God, our Creator.

Nevertheless, learning your child has special needs—whether you find out prior to or immediately after their birth, or a few months or years down the road—is difficult. Your love for your child instinctively wants them to be 'normal'. You don't want them to have to struggle. You don't want them to have to go through the experience of feeling different from the rest of the kids or to experience the loneliness often felt from being left out of so many things kids like to do. You don't want to see the hurt in their eyes and know their hearts are breaking when they are made fun of or ostracized by their peers.

What's more, you can't help worrying about how their condition or circumstances is going to affect your life and the lives of other family members. And then you start feeling guilty for feeling and thinking that way; making you even more anxious.

Am I right? You know I am. But the GREAT news is that it is perfectly normal and okay to feel and think these things—as long as you are near enough to Jesus to dump it all at His feet so that he can replace all of those things with what you need in order to do the very special job you have been given by God to do.

That's right—being given the responsibility of parenting a child with special needs is NOT a form of discipline or punishment. Instead, God is saying, "I have a special job for you because your heart's capacity to love and nurture is above and beyond what is normal. I created you with the ability to see beyond the obvious into the heart and soul of one of my children, so I need you to raise them up for me."

We see this truth in the Gospel of John, chapter nine, when Jesus heals a man who had been born blind. Jesus and His disciples were coming into a village when they saw the man, who was most likely begging in front of the marketplace or along the road that led into the village.

When the disciples saw that he was blind, they asked Jesus whether it was he or his parents whose sin had caused him to be born blind. (That's the punishment 'thing' I just mentioned.)

Jesus immediately replied that neither the sins of the man nor those of his parents had caused his blindness. And then in the next breath, Jesus added these words: Jesus answered, "Neither this man nor his parents sinned, but that the works of God should be revealed in him..." (John 9:3 NKJV)

Did you get that? The man's blindness wasn't a curse or punishment. He had been born blind so that he could be an instrument through which Jesus' holiness and power could be displayed. He was literally a partner in Jesus' ministry!

So while parenting a special-needs child maybe wasn't what you anticipated doing as a parent, and while you may feel completely overwhelmed and even terrified at the prospect of doing so, don't let these feelings rob your child of the joy he or she deserves to feel in your touch and see in your eyes that says, "I'm so glad you are mine." And whatever you do, don't let these feelings rob you of the joy you deserve to experience in becoming and being a parent and of the blessing of being God's partner in showing the world just how Holy and Mighty He is.

Bible Verses to Encourage You

And not only that, but we also glory in tribulations, knowing that tribulation produces perseverance; 4 and perseverance, character; and character, hope. ~Romans 5:3-4

And the Lord said unto him, who hath made man's mouth? or who maketh the dumb, or deaf, or the seeing, or the blind? have not I the Lord? ~Exodus 4:11

For thou hast possessed my reins: thou hast covered me in my mother's womb. I will praise thee; for I am fearfully and wonderfully made: marvelous are thy works; and that my soul knoweth right well. ~Psalm 139:13-14

Lo, children are an heritage of the Lord: and the fruit of the womb is his reward. ~Psalm 127:3

Chapter 2: Guarding Your Heart, Soul, Mind, and Strength

You can have all the joy, joy, joy, joy down in your heart, in your head, and bubbling up out of your soul imaginable but that won't erase the fact that parenting a special-needs child is hard work. It is physically exhausting, mentally and emotionally draining, time-consuming, and often times very, very lonely. I think it's safe to say that this is one of those things about which your grandma would say, "The most worthwhile jobs we do are the hardest jobs we do".

Because there is so much required of you, it is important that you take care of yourself. *Good* care of yourself. This is something many parents of special-needs children don't do a very well. Generally speaking, parents put the needs of their children in front of their own needs—as we should in many instances, but not *all*.

And when you take into consideration that the demands on your life because of the increased needs of your child…. I guess you could say that parents of special-needs children have some special needs of their own.

What you are about to read is a list of things you need to be doing for YOURSELF. Don't make excuses and the words "I can't" are not allowed—not even in your head or under your breath. Taking good care of yourself is key to doing your job to the best of your ability and key to knowing you, too, are fearfully and wonderfully made (Psalm 139).

1: Spend time in the Word daily

Ten or fifteen minutes spent reading the Bible each day is food for the soul, body, and mind. Don't just focus on the Psalms or the Gospels—books of the Bible that are usually viewed as the 'feel good' books of the Bible. While you *do* need to make them part of your Bible study, they shouldn't be the only part.

When you spend time in the books of history you become more grounded and sure of the fact that God does have a plan.

The books of Job and Ecclesiastes humble you and remind you that the most important things in life aren't things and that God really does have the whole world (including you and your child) in His hands.

The book of Esther gives us an extra dose of courage and reminds us that our ultimate purpose is to bring Glory to God through all we do and say.

The prophets don't spare words. They tell it like it is when it comes to reminding us that we are all sinners. But they are equally eloquent when it comes to reminding us of God's abundant love and mercy—love and mercy we can draw on every...single...day.

James and most of Paul's letters are the books that keep us on the straight and narrow. They define Christian character, warn us of the consequences for living outside of God's laws and expectations, and reaffirm the promises of heaven in all its glory when we abide in Jesus Christ.

Read God's Word. Apply it to your life. Let it speak to you. Let it change you.

2: Pray

One of the biggest concerns and complaints of parents with special-needs children is that they don't have many people they can talk to who really 'gets' it. Not on a regular basis, that is, because the parents who *do* 'get' it are as busy as they are. But God always hears and He is always available. No, He's not someone you can sit around the table with over a cup of coffee or someone you can chat with while you take a lap or two around the block.

But He *is* there, He *does* listen, and He *does* care.

You also need to know (or be reminded of the fact) that your conversations are not one-sided. God responds to you. He responds by:

- Telling the Holy Spirit what to say to you (Jon 16:13)
- Speaking to you through the Scriptures
- Providing answers through your conversations and interactions with others – Something called Confirmation.

In 1 Thessalonians 5:17 we are told to pray without ceasing. If you do that, you'll also be conversing with God nonstop.

3: Eat a healthy diet

God created our bodies to operate at optimum efficiency and capacity when we feed our bodies a steady diet of the food He created for us to eat. Meat, fruits, veggies, dairy products, grains...the things He created to fuel our bodies.

Sure there are exceptions—food allergies and personal tastes, for example. But for the most part you really need to make sure your diet consists primarily of foods free of chemicals, dyes, and processing.

If you are still looking for things like chips, blooming onions, mocha latte caramel coffee with an extra shot of caffeine, diet soda, and seven-layer lasagna on the list of best foods, you can stop. They aren't there. They never will be.

Eating a healthy diet keeps your body working the way it should. Your heart is healthier. Your body doesn't produce a lot of bad fat for you to carry around. You think more clearly. You reduce your risk of getting things like heart disease, diabetes, kidney failure, and bone and joint disorders due to carrying around too much weight. You have more energy. Your immune system does a better job of fighting off colds and the flu.

Question: What's not to like about the benefits of eating a healthy diet?

Answer: Nothing. So do it!

4: Get plenty of exercise

If your child has physical limitations that require you to bathe them, dress them, and help them move from one place to another, you are undoubtedly getting quite a bit of physical activity.

But that doesn't mean you don't need to get twenty minutes or so of walking, yoga, aerobics, or whatever else you like to do at least three days a week.

If at all possible, you should also set aside an hour or two each week for more rigorous exercise. A few possible options include: Water aerobics, tennis, volleyball, working out at the gym, swimming laps, or anything else you enjoy that gets your heart pumping.

The physical benefits of exercise go without saying and should be reason enough to make sure you get this time each week. But the physical benefits are just the tip of the proverbial iceberg. So what are the benefits?

- Exercise increases oxygen to the brain; helping you clear your head and think more rationally and clearly.

- Exercise releases endorphins. Endorphins are hormones that send messages to the brain that tell the brain to think positive thoughts. Endorphins also lessen our perception of pain. They intercept the signals from our nerves and send the message to the brain that it doesn't hurt as bad as 'all that'.
- Exercise keeps your weight in check and your heart healthy.
- Exercise gives you some much-deserved time off from your responsibilities as a parent. Even if it is only for a few minutes a day, it is worth it.
- Exercise boosts your immune system. This is actually one of the top two or three reasons parents of special-needs children take time to exercise.

- After all, when parents get sick (especially Mom) chaos at home can quickly ensue. So remember… "An ounce of prevention is worth a pound of cure".
- Some forms of exercise provide you with a social outlet. Even if you and a friend take several laps around the block or park, it still counts as time you can enjoy conversations without interruptions.

5: Date nights and marriage protection

Couples with children—no matter how many and no matter what their needs are—all run the risk of letting parenting, work, money-matters, and everything else push their marriage and its wellbeing to the backburner. But when you add the stresses of raising a special-needs child to the mix, the chances of this happening increase significantly.

The financial burdens that come from having a special-needs child are often very heavy to bear. The primary caregiver (usually Mom) doesn't have a lot of time to just sit and talk. She doesn't always have the luxury of prioritizing how her time is spent. That is usually done for her out of sheer necessity. That's why as parents of a special-needs child you need to make conscious and consistent effort to have couple time free of ANY talk about home, money, the kids, or anything else that pertains to your daily routine. You need to make a conscious effort to make romantic gestures and let your spouse know they are second only to God.

What? But...our child needs me to do.... Who has time for romance? And since my life pretty much revolves around making sure our kids are taken care of, there's not really much else to talk about.

Oh, but there is. There is plenty to talk about:

- Make plans for a weekend getaway…just the two of you
- Talk about an upcoming event at church
- Talk about some things you would like to make time to do for yourself
- Make plans for a family weekend
- Talk about current events
- Recall memories from your dating years and the early years of your marriage
- Talk about the reasons you love one another
- Talk about long-range goals for your marriage and family
- Talk about something funny you saw on television or at the grocery store
- Make a list of ideas of things you can do to keep your marriage fresh and thriving…and then start doing the things on that list

There are several other things you need to make sure you don't neglect to do in order to keep your marriage safe and fresh. These things include:

- Worshipping together.
- Serving together in your church and community.
- Letting your children see and hear you being (appropriately) affectionate with each other.
- Not allowing your children to play you against one another.
- Making sure you kiss each other good morning, hello, goodbye, and goodnight.
- Telling each other "I love you" every single day.
- Not neglecting your appearance—your 'Sunday best' isn't always necessary, but baggy pants, t-shirts, and a messy-hair-don't-care look doesn't say much about the way you feel about yourself.

- And if you don't care about yourself, it's hard for other people to do so.
- Taking care of your body.
- Showing an interest in your spouse's job (in and away from the home).
- Making their friends feel welcome in your home.
- Respecting their need for 'me' time and giving them that luxury.
- Making sure 'me' time and 'friend' time never add up to more than the time you spend with your spouse and your family.
- Living with the attitude of submission (for wives) and sacrificial love and leadership (for husbands) as directed in the New Testament book of Ephesians.

7: Fellowship

You need fellowship. You need to spend time with your peers; studying God's Word, socializing, enjoying recreational activities and outings, and just hanging out. Just being yourself.

While there is nothing wrong with part of this fellowship coming in the form of support groups or play groups with other parents of special-needs children, this should not be your *only* outlet. These groups are can be very beneficial—a lifeline for many of you—but you need to be able to fellowship in ways that address *your* needs and interests…not your child's.

Don't think this is being selfish. It's not. By giving yourself this time you are giving your family a better and you—an energized, more confident, refreshed you. So don't feel guilty about taking some time for a Bible study, a weekly game of golf or tennis, meeting up for coffee and fellowship, a book club, or some other group where you can share your passion for your hobby with others who feel the same.

The amount of time you allow yourself isn't a number that is set in stone. There is no magic number that guarantees your needs will be met. For some, an afternoon, evening, or possibly an entire day (or most of it, anyway) a week is doable. For others, though, an hour or two a week is a priceless and treasured gift that happens only with a great deal of planning, preparation, and help from others.

Speaking of help...

8: Ask for help

You can't do this on your own.
Physically...emotionally...mentally...you need help and support.

The help and support you receive can come from a number of different resources. Some of these resources exist solely for the purpose of helping parents of special-needs children and the children themselves. Other sources of help are people who love and care about you and want to be the hands and feet of Jesus in your life. And you need to let them do that.

Bobby and Shannon were the parents of six year-old twins and a three year-old born without hands—his arms stop just below his elbows. Bobby, Shannon, and all three children are completely comfortable with their life. Even the twins are a great help when it comes to feeding, dressing, and playing with their little brother.

But they are hesitant to leave their son in anyone's care other than his grandparents when they came to visit or the physical therapist they met with a couple of hours a week. So other than these two hours a week and four or five visits a year from grandparents, Bobby and Shannon took no time for just the two of them.

Friends from church have offered to take all three of the kids on numerous occasions, but Shannon always made an excuse. Thanks, but no thanks, was the message she conveyed. But then one day, a middle-aged woman at church asked Shannon a question that stopped her in her tracks. She asked, " Why do you insist on keeping people from doing what Jesus wants them to do?"

"Excuse me," Shannon asked back, somewhat offended. "What do you mean?"

"People in this church, including me, want to be part of your family and want you to be part of ours. We want to minister to your family, get to know you and your kids, let you know you have people who love and care about you. We want to live and love the way Jesus told us to, but you won't let us," was the woman's answer.

Shannon didn't know what to say. She'd never thought about it like that before. She was so focused on not wanting to appear to be a charity case or give people a reason to think they needed to feel sorry for them and their son, that she had completely forgotten that Jesus calls us to love and serve one another. This woman was right! By not accepting their offers for help and fellowship, they were robbing these people of opportunities to be like Jesus. And what's more, they were robbing themselves of the blessings that come with being a part of a family of believers.

From that day on Shannon and Bobby were more than happy to take people up on their offers to babysit so they could have date nights. And they were equally happy to return the favor by doing the same for other young families in the church. Josephine (the woman who talked to Shannon) and her husband became surrogate grandparents to their children, and relationships were built that will undoubtedly last a lifetime.

Today Shannon and Bobby are the parents for four and grandparents to two. They are also in charge of a parent's night out ministry at their church, because they know what it is like to need help AND they know how important it is for others to be able to offer it.

Besides your church family, other possible resources for help include:

- Healthcare agencies
- Playgroups for children with physical disabilities
- Daycare facilities that cater to children with special needs
- Friends and neighbors
- Support groups (for emotional and mental help you need)

9: Me time

In addition to the time you spend with just your spouse and time spent with your friends and peers, you need to have a few minutes of 'me' time every day. Thirty minutes or so each day to do whatever you want to do by yourself. Take a walk. Soak in the bathtub. Read a book. Bake cookies. Shoot some hoops. Watch television without interruption. Surf the web. Catch up on social media. Do your nails. Take a nap. Whatever you enjoy doing…do it.

The purpose of this time of solitude is to allow you to clear your head and not think about anyone or anything but yourself and what you are doing. This is your time to dream, plan, rest, relax, and even be a bit selfish.

Taking this time each day is so important. Knowing you have this time to look forward to each day helps you keep things in the proper perspective. It prevents you from feeling like you've lost your identity as an individual.

You are God's child. You are a spouse. You are a parent. You are an instrument of God's plan. Your body is the temple of the Holy Spirit. You cannot be and do these things if you are not practicing good self-care, so do it. It is your duty to yourself, your family, and to your God.

Embrace Your Special Needs Child, Prayer, and Parenting
Bible Verses to Encourage You

It is vain for you to rise up early, to sit up late, to eat the bread of sorrows: for so he giveth his beloved sleep. ~Psalm 127:2

*I will both lie down in peace, and sleep;
For You alone, O Lord, make me dwell in safety. ~Psalm 4:8*

For I have satiated the weary soul, and I have replenished every sorrowful soul. ~Jeremiah 31:25

*There remaineth therefore a rest to the people of God. For he that is entered into his rest, he also hath ceased from his own works, as God did from His.
~Hebrews 4:9-10*

Chapter 3: True Love is Devoid of All Pride

Every parent's desire is to make their child's life good, happy, pleasant, and as carefree as possible. And why not? Isn't that just part of what loving someone is all about? But when you have a child with special needs, your quest to give these things to your child usually comes with a few (or a lot) more challenges.

Every parent is charged by God with the task of keeping their children safe and healthy, providing them with food, clothing, and shelter, and loving them unconditionally; nurturing and cherishing them for the treasure they are. Additionally, parents are responsible for raising their children to:

- Learn to be confident and comfortable with who they are
- Know that we are to be God-pleasers…not people-pleasers
- Recognize sin for what it is and rise above it

- To strive to achieve their goals and dreams

But again, children with special needs have to work a little harder to get the job done, and as their parent, *you* have to work a little harder to help them. Your success in doing so depends on your ability to set aside any prideful feelings you have—consciously or subconsciously.

Denial is not uncommon when you first learn that your child has special needs. These feelings are not necessarily evidence of shame or embarrassment. More often than not they stem from guilt, concern, and apprehension.

- Did I do something…or not do something that caused this?
- Will my child be able to enjoy at least some of the things a child should?
- Can I be the parent my child needs and deserves?

The reason for the feelings isn't necessarily important. What *is* important is that you set them aside for the sake of everyone involved. Don't let pride keep you from dong what is best for your child.

Early intervention

Denial has been the reason for many children's conditions and disabilities to go undiagnosed as soon as they could and should be. If your child isn't diagnosed as having special needs, then the problem isn't really there, right? Wrong! Early intervention often makes the difference in how severely their disability affects their life (and yours) and the degree to which they can function.

Parents, pretending or burying your head in the sand accomplishes nothing good. So don't deny your child every chance possible to be high-functioning and/or to receive therapy that allows them to be more mobile and independent. Get help at the first sign that a problem exists.

Your pediatrician will be able to connect you with available resources and information for your particular situation. Make use of them.

Living realistically

Once you know what your child's condition is and what their needs are and will be you need to listen intently and carefully to those who can point you in the right direction to get you and your child the help available to you. When meeting with therapists, doctors, and anyone else involved in your child's care, you might not always like what you hear. Sometimes parents feel the plan of action isn't aggressive enough. Some feel it is too aggressive. And some think the medical community is too pessimistic in their outlook. These are the parents that believe if their child tries hard enough they can overcome their disability.

EXAMPLE: Jared's mom was thoroughly convinced that putting her son in a classroom for special-needs students that he would never reach his full potential. She believed that if he was in a traditional classroom setting he would work harder to be on a level 'playing field' with the rest of the class.

The problem with this line of thinking is that by putting expectations on Jared he simply cannot meet makes him feel bad about himself and causes him to doubt his ability to succeed. It's like giving a five year-old keys to the car and expecting them to be able to drive.

Your child has enough to deal with because of their special needs. Don't add to that by trying to make them someone they are not and by insinuating that you are ashamed of them or that who they are is not reason enough to love them with your whole heart. Accept the fact that they have limitations. Accept what those limitations are. Put them in a position to excel to the best of their ability. Celebrate their accomplishments. Love them for who they are.

Be your child's advocate and biggest fan

Today's children are only the second or third generation of children to not be hidden away or ignored just because they have special needs. Prior to this, children with special needs were considered to be disposable and less valuable than their 'normal' peers. Children with special needs and disabilities were often placed in institutions where they did little more than exist. Others were kept at home, but were not allowed to go to school and had little or no social interaction. Think: Boo Radley in *To Kill a Mockingbird*.

Thankfully, though, not every parent 'back then' thought or felt that way...

Neal and Bonita knew something was wrong with their second-born son, Gary, before he turned six months old. He wasn't meeting the developmental milestones for babies his age.

But in those days and in their small town, it wasn't easy to get a correct diagnosis. When they did, the words they heard were MULTIPLE SCLEROSIS.

Neal and Bonita were encouraged to put Gary in a 'home' where he could live out his days (which they were told would be less than twenty years) peacefully and out of the harsh and unaccepting public eye. But they didn't want to put their son away. They knew God didn't make a mistake when he made Gary. They knew he was as treasured and loved as anyone else God created. They also knew that every child with special needs was one of God's precious treasures, too. So with nothing but a determination and passion for wanting to help Gary and others like him to reach their full potential, Neal and Bonita recruited teachers and people who practiced a trade to work in what would now be called a sheltered workshop.

Gary is now an eighty year-old man who has never walked on his own, never ran, played catch, or spoken a word that is understandable by an 'untrained' ear. But he *has* appeared before three different presidents of the United States to champion for the rights of people with disabilities, gone to Europe to compete in the Special Olympics, won multiple gold and silver medals in the same, accumulated dozens of bowling trophies, and encouraged countless people just by being himself. But these things were possible only because his parents were his biggest fans and they championed for him with relentless energy, passion, and love.

Don't let anyone make your child feel worthless and unlovable. Believe in them and do whatever you can to make sure they are given every possible and feasible opportunity to reach their full potential.

Embrace Your Special Needs Child, Prayer, and Parenting
Bible Verses to Encourage You

For I know the thoughts that I think toward you, saith the Lord, thoughts of peace, and not of evil, to give you a future and a hope. ~Jeremiah 29:11

Now unto Him that is able to do exceeding abundantly above all that we ask or think, according to the power that worketh in us... ~Ephesians 3:20

For we are His workmanship, created in Christ Jesus unto good works, which God hath before ordained that we should walk in them. ~Ephesians 2:10

Chapter 4: Overcoming the Educational Obstacles

Back in the day there was an ad campaign targeting high schoolers in an effort to convince them to pursue a college education. The campaign's slogan was, "A mind is a terrible thing to waste". And it's true, a mind *is* a terrible thing to waste—and that means your child, too.

Depending on where you live, your child's school may or may not be equipped to offer your child the educational resources they need and deserve. This is not something you should waste time being angry or bitter about. In most cases the lack of resources is due to a lack of money and/or a lack of qualified teachers in the district—neither of which will be changed by your anger or bitterness. Instead, be pro-active and take matters into your own hands. Instead of wasting your time and energy, put it to use by either becoming the resources your child needs or by going beyond the walls of the school to get them.

Here are some possible ways you might do that:

Depending on your child's special needs you might consider homeschooling your child. Or better yet, consider forming a homeschool coop with other special need's parents. This has proven to be especially helpful to both parents and students with needs such as dyslexia, mild autism, sensory problems, auditory processing disorder, and a variety of delayed development issues. Educating your child in this type of environment allows them to:

- Learn in a less congested environment with fewer distractions and risks of over-stimulation and more personalized attention
- Feel safer and more accepted among their peers
- Receive instruction and training at a pace and in a format that will allow them to thrive and excel

As for parents, working together shares the workload, provides a community of support and encouragement, and it allows you to know you are giving your child the learning environment most conducive to their learning style and capabilities.

Hire a tutor. Homeschooling on any level is not always possible. And quite frankly, it is not always the best route to take. Depending on your child's needs and the resources they have available in their school, you may find that by hiring a tutor your child will be able to stay on course with the mainstream student population. You don't need to go through a professional service to find a good tutor, though. Retired teachers, teachers who have opted to stay home with their own children, but who are willing to tutor a few hours a week, or college students in need of extra money are all great resources. A tutor gives your child the one-on-one they so often need to get them over the hump and to give them the moral support and encouragement to keep trying.

Specialized schools are available in some areas—usually large cities. These are somewhat expensive, however, but *do* offer the best in special-needs education. If you live near one of these schools don't let the price tag scare you. Funding is sometimes available through scholarship programs or organizations to aid and assist children with special needs.

Public schooling is free and available to children with mild to moderately-severe special needs. Many public schools have excellent programs for children with learning disabilities and a staff of loving, caring, and dedicated teachers. Often time's public schools also offer and allow personal aides or assistants for special-needs students. The job of a personal aide/assistant is to be their student's constant companion throughout the day; assisting them in whatever ways they need assistance.

Some of the things they might do include:

- Reading to them if they cannot read but can comprehend
- Signing for the deaf
- Writing for those that cannot write but are fully able to comprehend and can speak the answers
- Feeding and other personal care

No matter what educational obstacles you encounter or what path you choose for your child, remember...a mind is a terrible thing to waste.

Embrace Your Special Needs Child, Prayer, and Parenting
Bible Verses to Encourage You

How much better is it to get wisdom than gold! and to get understanding rather to be chosen than silver! ~Proverbs 16:16

*Take firm hold of instruction, do not let go;
Keep her, for she is your life.
~Proverbs 4:13*

Give instruction to a wise man, and he will be yet wiser: teach a just man, and he will increase in learning. ~Proverbs 9:9

Chapter 5: We Are Family

When asked what challenges a special-needs child brings to the dynamics of a family, the answers are all over the map.

- "I don't think of my child's needs as something that challenges our family," one parent said. "Being a family means seeing one another as equally valuable and loving one another for who we are. So if who we are, is someone who needs help eating or who cannot play ball, then so be it."
- "I find myself working harder than I really need to sometimes to make things equal for my kids. Sometimes I feel guilty about spending more time with my daughter because of her needs, but then God reminds me that not having to do those things for my boys is a good thing."

- "It is challenging. My now-seven year-old was three when an accident left her with some physical disabilities and mild learning disabilities. I was expecting our second child at the time, so adjusting to all the changes in our routine and life in general really did keep me from enjoying my new baby. I am constantly second-guessing myself in regards to how good a mom I am to each of them."
- "I leave for work every morning knowing my wife is on a non-stop schedule. I feel guilty for being gone so much, but our son's medical expenses are over the top. We'll never be able to see the light at the end of the tunnel. We would like to have another child, but don't know how in the world we could handle two.

- We want to know what it's like to parent a child that doesn't need round the clock care (or close to it). We want to know what it's like to go to our kid's ball game or dance recital. Is that so bad or wrong?"
- We have two boys in school and our four year-old son is low-functioning autistic. The six and nine year old boys are great with him at home, but I've noticed lately they get embarrassed when Judson acts out in public and they say things like, "Can't you just take us and Mom and Judson stay home?" Or "Judson can't do that, so why does he have to come?" I know some of that is natural, but right now I'm really struggling with how to teach my boys to love their brother for who he is and to love him like they love each other."

I could say all sorts of things on how I feel or what I think on how to handle the possible challenges a special-needs child can bring to your family. But what I think and how I feel aren't important. What is important is what God has to say on the subject of family unity…regardless of the physical, mental, or emotional issues that might be present. So take a few minutes to let God's Word soak into your heart and mind. Share these verses with your spouse, your children, and even your extended family members in an effort to remind them that we are ALL created in the image of God and are ALL equally loved and valued by him.

Bible Verses to Encourage You

Love suffers long and is kind; love does not envy; love does not parade itself, is not puffed up; does not behave rudely, does not seek its own, is not provoked, thinks no evil; does not rejoice in iniquity, but rejoices in the truth; bears all things, believes all things, hopes all things, endures all things ~1 Corinthians 13:4-7 (NKJV)

We love him, because he first loved us.
~1 John 4:19

Better is a dry morsel with quietness,
Than a house full of feasting with strife.
~Proverbs 17:1

For as we have many members in one body, but all the members do not have the same function, so we, being many, are one body in Christ, and individually members of one another. ~Romans 12:4-5

For the body is not one member, but many. If the foot shall say, because I am not the hand, I am not of the body; is it therefore not of the body? And if the ear shall say, because I am not the eye, I am not of the body; is it therefore not of the body? If the whole body were an eye, where were the hearing? If the whole were hearing, where were the smelling? But now hath God set the members every one of them in the body, as it hath pleased him. ~1 Corinthians 12:15-18

Chapter 6: Let Your "Light" Shine

Remember reading about Neal and Bonita and how they refused to stifle their son, Gary's potential in time when that was the norm for kids like Gary? Thankfully things are much different today.

Today parks have playgrounds for children with even the most severe disabilities.

Today public buildings have rams and entryways that are accessible to people in a wheelchair.

Today public restrooms are equipped with facilities with enough room to maneuver around in and with sinks, toilets, etc. placed at the right height.

Today even campground shower houses have wheelchair-accessible showers.

Today parking lots provide spaces for vehicles with special-needs drivers or passengers.

Today special-needs children can grow up to be special-needs adults who contribute to society in a positive manner by working, volunteering, and just living life to the fullest.

All of these things are definitely improvements over what used to be, but that doesn't mean life for families of special-needs children is not without its share of obstacles in their communities and their social lives.

When it comes to meeting and overcoming the challenges of special-needs children and their families in the community and on the social 'scene', you need to respond the same way you should when it comes to your child's education. You need to be a pro-active advocate instead of an angry, bitter parent. And the best way to do this is to help the world see what an amazing and precious person your child is.

Proverbs 31:8 (NKJV) says: *Open your mouth for the speechless, In the cause of all who are appointed to die.* So do it! Open your mouth, use your hands to open doors, your feet to walk through them, and your mind to think of ways to help your child be a part of the world around them. Don't hide their light under a basket. Let them shine for all those around them to see...and be blessed.

- Attend church and let your child be involved in the youth program to the extent they are capable of. Be willing to act as a chaperone for youth events so that your child can participate.
- Volunteer with your child. Taking their specific needs into consideration, consider participating in walk-a-thons (or wheel-a-thons, if necessary). Fill shoe boxes with gifts for other children. Ring the Salvation Army bells. Hand out personal care bags to the homeless. Visit a nursing home together.
- Join a play group.

- Visit the park on a regular basis.
- Enroll your child in swimming lessons, bowling lessons, or some other type of activity they are capable of participating in. *Many of these activities/lessons offer special lessons for children with various handicaps.
- Join 4-H, scouts, or another similar type of organization.
- Go to the weekly story hour at your library.
- Participate in free movie nights, craft-making events, kid-friendly lectures and demonstrations, etc. offered in your community.
- Go for ice cream or an occasional dinner at a favorite family pizza place or restaurant.
- Get them involved with Special Olympics.

The "Bible Verses to Encourage You" segments in previous chapters have already listed Exodus 4:11 and Psalm 139:13-14, but I want us to look at them again because they are important reminders to everyone that God creates each of us in his image and with a distinct set of purposes in mind. Special-needs children are not mistakes. God doesn't make mistakes. Special-needs children are special-*purposes* children and as their parents you need to help them accomplish those purposes in this world.

Bible Verses to Encourage You

And the Lord said unto him, who hath made man's mouth? or who maketh the dumb, or deaf, or the seeing, or the blind? have not I the Lord? ~Exodus 4:11

For thou hast possessed my reins: thou hast covered me in my mother's womb. I will praise thee; for I am fearfully and wonderfully made: marvelous are thy works; and that my soul knoweth right well. ~Psalm 139:13-14

But indeed, O man, who are you to reply against God? Will the thing formed say to Him who formed it, "Why have you made me like this?" ~Romans 9:20

Chapter 7: Dealing With Special Social and Communication Needs

Children with social and communication special needs are those with autism, Asperger, and ADHD (as well as a few others). But then you already know that, don't you? You know that your child has difficulties interacting socially and communicating their thoughts and needs.

The severity of these conditions varies widely from person to person. In some children it is a matter of controlling their intake of certain foods and providing them with a structured environment so that they don't feel (and act) like a loose cannon. But for others, the problem is much more intense. Some children cannot speak or communicate on any level. Some children cannot handle even slight changes in their routine without becoming unsettled and sometime nearly impossible to manage or console. But again, you already know these things.

What you don't know...or need to be reminded of is that neither you nor your child is alone in the struggles you are facing to deal with life as you know it. God is ever-present.

His presence is visible in the words of the Bible:

He healeth the broken in heart, and bindeth up their wounds. ~Psalm 147:3

It is of the Lord's mercies that we are not consumed, because His compassions fail not. They are new every morning: great is thy faithfulness. The Lord is my portion, saith my soul; therefore will I hope in Him. The Lord is good unto them that wait for Him, to the soul that seeketh him. ~Lamentations 3:22-25

But God commendeth His love toward us, in that, while we were yet sinners, Christ died for us. ~Romans 5:8

Another means by which God proves His presence is in providing resources and counsel for you and your child. Because God has worked through others, we know that parents of children with autism and ADHD can help their child when they:

- Provide a consistent routine and schedule for their child
- Make home a safe, fun, and hazard-free place to be
- Make time for fun; doing things THEY enjoy doing
- Reward positive behavior
- Discover their child's triggers for tantrums and melt-downs and then take necessary actions and precautions
- Know the child's sensitivities (smell, sound, etc.) and try to avoid them or forewarn them
- Concentrate on the child's strengths; allowing them to achieve and excel

- Teach older children to use public transportation, tech gadgets, and other helps in order to be more independent
- Teach them to respect themselves
- Teach them to love, honor, and obey the LORD

Parents of children with Asperger's can help their children by:

- Help your child practice appropriate reactions to common social situations at home so they can learn without feeling judged or on display.
- Teach your children the meaning of common phrases that aren't meant to be taken literally, since many children with Asperger's are quite literal. Example: Telling a child with Asperger's that he is silly will often get this type of response: "I'm not silly, I'm Max."

- Give your child a safety phrase—something to say that will alert you that they are feeling anxious and scared and unsure of how to respond or react.
- Prevent situations when possible rather than try to cure them after the fact.
- Plan ahead and keep your child informed of what they can expect. Surprises and the unexpected are NOT enjoyable to them.
- Don't argue with your child. Negotiate or end the conversation until both of you are better able to communicate rationally.
- Let them 'run with' the things that interest them and don't try to squelch their methods of imaginary play.

Whatever level of function your child has, remember this: They are precious in God's sight and are significant to His plan.

Chapter 8: Dealing With Special Neurological Needs

In an effort to encourage you to stay the course and keep things in their proper perspective, I want to offer you a list of tips and suggestions for dealing with the special needs of your child in a way that will benefit them and the rest of your family. Remember: Every child deserves to know, beyond a doubt, that the only reason you *need* to love them is because they are yours—that that's enough to merit your unconditional love.

Keeping that in mind, here are some things you can do to help your child with sensory processing disorder:

- Slow down. A lot of times children will be able to accept and enjoy new experiences if they are allowed to approach them at a slower pace.

- Give them space. Again, they need time to adjust to their surroundings and assess them in their own way.
- Keep things as visual as possible, as kids with sensory disorders are usually calmed by what they can see.
- Keep a bag full of items to distract your kids from sensory overload handy at ALL times.
- Be sensitive to their thoughts, feelings, and needs. Don't force things on them that aren't necessary.
- Introduce new sights, sounds, textures, and smells in a positive manner. Teach them to try something new, but let their response be the indicator of how far to take it.
- A therapy or specialized play group can be beneficial. Sometimes positive peer pressure works for the good of your child.

Children with auditory processing disorder:

- Should receive instructions in short, simple sentences. One step at a time.
- Should always be spoken to when facing them and when you are sure you have their attention.
- Keep things as visual as possible. Use chore charts, to-do lists, etc.
- Ask questions like: "Do you understand?" "Do you know what you are supposed to do?" "What did I just say to you?" Ask these questions in a loving, affirmative tone—not one that is condescending and degrading.
- Provide your child with simple puzzles, I-spy books, and toys that produce visible results.

Children with Tourette's and Epilepsy:

- Make sure your child takes their medication on schedule.
- Have regular medical checkups and evaluations.
- Make sure everyone in the family, teachers, and caregivers know what to do in the event of a seizure.
- Educate those who live and work with your child on the facts about Tourette's, Epilepsy, or other neurological disorder.
- Remember that the vast majority of children with Tourette's and Epilepsy have no mental or emotional disabilities. They are what society considers high-functioning children.
- Children with Epilepsy should always wear helmets when riding a bike or skating.

- Never allow an epileptic child to swim alone or be left alone in the tub. Older children should not be allowed to take a bath...showers only.
- Make sure your child has a medical alert bracelet or necklace on in the event they require emergency care and you are not with them. This will allow those around them to get the help your child needs.

REMEMBER: Awareness and knowledge are your child's two best allies when it comes to living with and thriving in spite of their special needs.

Embrace Your Special Needs Child, Prayer, and Parenting
Bible Verses to Encourage You

You also, as living stones, are being built up a spiritual house, a holy priesthood, to offer up spiritual sacrifices acceptable to God through Jesus Christ. 1 Peter 2:5 (NKJV)

Be anxious for nothing, but in everything by prayer and supplication, with thanksgiving, let your requests be made known to God; and the peace of God, which surpasses all understanding, will guard your hearts and minds through Christ Jesus. ~Philippians 4:6-7

*Take heed that ye despise not one of these little ones; for I say unto you, that in heaven **their** angels do always behold the face of my Father which is in heaven. ~Matthew 18:10*

Chapter 9: Dealing with Genetic and Physical Special Needs

Among the most common physical and genetic problems facing parents of children with special needs include: cystic fibrosis, multiple sclerosis, cerebral palsy, downs syndrome, congenital birth defects of the vital organs or limbs, dyslexia, and muscular dystrophy.

There are of course, less common and even rare forms of these types of diseases and disorders including, dwarfism and SMA (spinal muscular atrophy)—to name just a few. And then there are those families dealing with special needs resulting from accidental injuries and problems resulting from the birth mother's abuse of drugs and alcohol.

No matter what the cause of the defect, disease, or injury, the fact remains that a child needs and deserves to enjoy the highest quality of life possible. Therefore, it is the wise and caring parent who makes the most of every opportunity and resource to help make that happen. You can be that parent when you:

- No matter what your child's special needs are, make sure everyone who lives with and spends time with your child on a regular basis knows what your child's condition is, what their needs are, has a working knowledge of how to meet those needs, and knows what to do in an emergency as well as how to do it.
- Make sure your child receives regular checkups and evaluations by their doctor and specialists.
- Make sure your child gets adequate rest, exercise (to the best of their ability), and social and intellectual stimulation and interaction.

- Make sure your child is eating a healthy and nutritious diet. Make this a family thing. For example: If your child is diabetic, don't make them feel deprived and different by keeping candy in the house for everyone else. Make it a special treat for everyone—even your diabetic on occasion.
- Be your child's advocate by taking whatever steps are necessary to ensure they receive the education they deserve and the assistance they need to reach their full potential.
- Do your homework. Stay up on the news concerning available resources for your child.

- Realize there are some things your child simply cannot do. When this happens you need to remember two things: 1) don't make your other children miss out on things. Let them enjoy the life they have been given. And 2) don't make a big deal out of it. Instead, focus on the things they *can* do and let them give those things 100%.

Children with Downs's Syndrome

- Embrace and enjoy their loving, affectionate nature.
- Encourage them to participate in social activities.
- Make sure they are receiving the best possible balance of mainstream classroom learning and classes targeted to meet their special needs. Downs kids are not dumb. They just need help learning how to express and use what they know.

- Parents of children with downs need to make exercise and healthy eating a priority to combat their tendency to be overweight and have heart problems.

Children with mobility needs

- Take your child for regular medical checkups and evaluations. Most mobility diseases and defects are progressive in nature; meaning they only get worse over time. You and your child need to know what is going on inside their body in order to meet their changing needs.
- Establish a regular routine for physical therapy. Movement of the right kind is essential for maintaining a quality of life for your child.
- Make sure your home is fully accessible to them. No child should feel unwelcome or in the way in their own home.

- Make sure your home is a safe place for your child. Loose rugs, exposed cords, and furniture that is unsteady can be hazardous.
- Equip your home in such a way that your child can grow into an independent young person. Make sure they can access the microwave and stovetop. Make sure the refrigerator opens in the direction necessary for them to be able to reach things easily. Make sure light switches are reachable. Lower the rods and shelves in their closet. Install a shower or tub to accommodate their needs with minimal or no assistance.

- Provide forms of exercise and entertainment they can enjoy at home: a swing set to accommodate their needs, a hot tub (ONLY with adult supervision), fuse ball, games with little or no physical movement required (trivia, etc.), audio books, and special instruments that will allow them to work the computer, and telephone.
- Take family outings that are wheelchair-friendly. Most state and national parks and sites are, as well as city parks, theaters, and amusement parks.

Children with genetic and other physical limitations

Genetic abnormalities can show themselves physically, mentally, or emotionally. The degree to which they show themselves also varies widely; ranging from things like dyslexia to an inability to speak or breathe without the assistance of a machine.

Because there are so many different forms or levels of special needs your child might have because of these things, it is important that you educate yourself as much as possible in regards to:

- The particulars of your child's needs and condition
- The resources available to you and your child
- What you can and cannot expect in the way of progression or digression
- What you should and shouldn't expect of your child
- How to properly care for your child
- How to help your child reach their full potential

When it's all is said and done, the most important thing you can remember as the parent of a special-needs child is that Jesus loves the little children - ALL the little children of the world – And that means Your Child too.

Embrace Your Special Needs Child, Prayer, and Parenting
Bible Verses to Encourage You

Lo, children are a heritage of the Lord: and the fruit of the womb is His reward.
~Psalm 127:3

Behold the fowls of the air: for they sow not, neither do they reap, nor gather into barns; yet your heavenly Father feedeth them. Are ye not much better than they? ~Matthew 6:26

for I was hungry and you gave Me food; I was thirsty and you gave Me drink; I was a stranger and you took Me in; I was naked and you clothed Me; I was sick and you visited Me; I was in prison and you came to Me. "Then the righteous will answer Him, saying, 'Lord, when did we see You hungry and feed You, or thirsty and give You drink? When did we see You a stranger and take You in, or naked and clothe You? Or when did we see You sick, or in prison, and come to You?' And the King will answer and say to them, **'Assuredly, I say to you, inasmuch as you did it to one of the least of these My brethren, you did it to Me.'.** *~Matthew 25:35-40*

Chapter 10: Your Not-So-Secret Secret Thoughts

As the parent of a special-needs child you have thoughts and feelings parents of other kids don't have. You think:

- Why my child? Why don't they get to run and play? Why can't they enjoy something as simple as licking an ice cream cone or sloshing through a mud puddle in their bare feet? Why do they have to be the one kids make fun of and shy away from?
- Why doesn't God answer my prayers to heal my child? He healed all those other people in the Bible?
- If I hear the term 'short bus', 'retard', or 'freak' one more time I'm going to explode all over whoever says it.

- I just wish I could have one day that was the kind of normal most people have.
- I know they say it's not my fault, but...but...is it...maybe?

And yes, some of you have even thought:

- If we wouldn't have had this to deal with, our marriage would have survived.
- It's not fair to my other children for me to have to devote so much of myself to their sibling.
- My husband or wife and I are never going to know what it's like to be just the two of us.
- What's going to happen to him/her when we can no longer take care of him/her? Who will take over?
- I'm so tired I don't know if I can do this again tomorrow.

You are only human, so it is natural for you to become weary, worried, and worn down. But the great news is—the news you *have to hold tight to*—is that you don't have to remain weary, worried, and worn down. God the Father, Jesus the Son, and the Holy Spirit are here to help. They are here to take these things from you and replace them with rest, peace, and hope.

As we close out our 'time' together, I want to leave you with some final words of encouragement from the scripture. My prayer is that these words will inspire you to be thankful for and mindful of the fact that you have been chosen by God to care for and rise up one of his extra-special children.

God bless you abundantly!

Bible Verses to Encourage You

Casting down arguments and every high thing that exalts itself against the knowledge of God, bringing every thought into captivity to the obedience of Christ; ~2 Corinthians 10:5

Finally, brethren, whatever things are true, whatever things are noble, whatever things are just, whatever things are pure, whatever things are lovely, whatever things are of good report, if there is any virtue and if there is anything praiseworthy—meditate on these things. ~Philippians 4:8

I beseech you therefore, brethren, by the mercies of God, that you present your bodies a living sacrifice, holy, acceptable to God, which is your reasonable service. And do not be conformed to this world, but be transformed by the renewing of your mind, that you may prove what is that good and acceptable and perfect will of God.~Romans 12:1-2

Embrace Your Special Needs Child, Prayer, and Parenting

Prayer

Your No. 1 Prayer Book to Learn To Be
A Strong Christian Prayer Warrior That Prays With
Powerful Prayers in The War Room To Overcome And
Defeat The Enemy

By: Patrick Baldwin

Disclaimer

This book is a guide to help you strengthen your prayer life – it is not intended to guarantee that God will answer your prayers. Often times when God doesn't answer our prayers it is in fact an answer to prayers. Yet not too many of us realize this reality, we feel if God doesn't answer our prayers something's wrong and we often question – why? The truth of the matter is we may never know the why here on this side of heaven, but rest in the promises of God for He is faithful and just to take you from glory to glory and that He will direct your steps along the way as you continue to pray. God does not forsake His children but at times chastises them much like a tree in need of pruning. It doesn't always feel good and it's not always pleasant but most assuredly we know we can trust in God no matter what.

Unfortunately in today's society I have to put this disclaimer in this book so everyone has a clear understanding that I make no promise, guarantee, or assurance whether directly or indirectly that God will answer any of your prayers – that is completely and totally at the sole discretion of Almighty God, the Alpha and Omega, the great I am.

Furthermore it should be completely understood as previously mentioned that often times when we pray and we don't see God answering our prayers God is in fact answering our prayers for He knows the things that you have need of even before you ask. This is a critical concept to understand for we may pray an error or contrary to God's will for life but thanks be to God who leads us and guides us despite our ignorance.

Preface

Prayer, along with the written Word (the Bible) is the most valuable tool we have when it comes to formulating a personal relationship with The Lord. The reason these two things are so essential can be summed up in one word—communication. It not only allows us to hear God, but communication is a two-way street. And prayer is the 'street' that allows us to communicate back to God.

Prayer is also the most misused, misunderstood, and un-used resource we have available to us. God created us in His image. His image! Do you understand what that means? It means we are as like God as any aspect of creation can be. It means we are special. It means God very much desires to have a relationship with us—one that is deeply personal. It means He will listen and answer our prayers when we pray because of His desire to be close to us.

You don't ignore your spouse, your children, your friends, or your boss when they talk to you, do you? Of course not! You also expect them to listen to you when you have something to say. So why do you think it should be any different with God? The answer to that question is this: It shouldn't be. Your willingness to talk to God and to have Him talk to you should be even greater than it is with the other relationships you have in your life.

The purpose of this book is to help you achieve that goal. By looking at what prayer is, how to pray, what to pray for, and when to pray, you will hopefully become more equipped and fully aware of what it means to pray to God and overcome and defeat the spiritual enemy.

Chapter 1: What is Prayer?

Prayer is conversation between you and God. It is both speaking and listening. You speak. God listens. God speaks. You listen.

You speak

Prayer is the time you spend talking to God about the cares and concerns of your heart. It is the time you tell Him the desires of your heart. It is time spent praising God for being His amazing, holy, and wonderful self. It is time spent confessing your sins and asking God's forgiveness. It is time spent talking to God on behalf of family, friends, your church, our government, our military, missionaries, and whoever or whatever else concerns you.

God listens

God listens to each and every word we say. He even listens to our thoughts. Philippians 4:6 says, *Be careful for nothing; but in every thing by prayer and supplication with thanksgiving let your requests be made known unto God.* Did you get that? We can (and should) go to God about everything.

God listened to Elijah when he questioned God's decision to allow the widow's son to die. Once more, God gave Elijah what he asked for: *And he cried unto the Lord, and said, O Lord my God, hast thou also brought evil upon the widow with whom I sojourn, by slaying her son? And he stretched himself upon the child three times, and cried unto the Lord, and said, O Lord my God, I pray thee, let this child's soul come into him again. And the Lord heard the voice of Elijah; and the soul of the child came into him again, and he revived.* (1 Kings 17:20-22)

God listened to Mordecai when he prayed that God would intervene and save the Jewish race from annihilation at the hand of Haman (Esther 4:1).

God listened to David when he asked God to forgive him for his sins of adultery and conspiracy for murder. David's prayer asking forgiveness is one of the most beautiful of all the psalms...

Have mercy upon me, O God, according to thy lovingkindness: according unto the multitude of thy tender mercies blot out my transgressions. Wash me throughly from mine iniquity, and cleanse me from my sin. For I acknowledge my transgressions: and my sin is ever before me. Against thee, thee only, have I sinned, and done this evil in thy sight: that thou mightest be justified when thou speakest, and be clear when thou judgest...

Purge me with hyssop, and I shall be clean: wash me, and I shall be whiter than snow. Make me to hear joy and gladness; that the bones which thou hast broken may rejoice. Hide thy face from my sins, and blot out all mine iniquities. Create in me a clean heart, O God; and renew a right spirit within me. Cast me not away from thy presence; and take not thy holy spirit from me. Restore unto me the joy of thy salvation; and uphold me with thy free spirit. (Psalm 51:1- 4 and 7-12)

God listened to Jesus when He asked God to forgive those who were responsible for His death when He said, *"Then said Jesus, Father, forgive them; for they know not what they do." (Luke 23:34)*

God speaks

When we pray, we're not the only ones doing the talking. God does plenty of talking when we pray. No, we don't audibly hear God's voice like Abraham, Moses, Jonah, and numerous others did normally.

But we hear God in that little voice that speaks to our heart and to our mind; telling us to do what we know is right and good. God's voice is the voice that warns us against sin and encourages us to go in the direction He created us to go.

Abraham's servant prayed to God; asking Him to provide the right woman for him to take home for Isaac to marry...

And he said O Lord God of my master Abraham, I pray thee, send me good speed this day, and shew kindness unto my master Abraham. Behold, I stand here by the well of water; and the daughters of the men of the city come out to draw water: And let it come to pass, that the damsel to whom I shall say,

Let down thy pitcher, I pray thee, that I may drink; and she shall say, Drink, and I will give thy camels drink also: let the same be she that thou hast appointed for thy servant Isaac; and thereby shall I know that thou hast shewed kindness unto my master. (Genesis 24:12-14)

God spoke to this man by giving him exactly what he asked for—a clear and definite answer as to the girl he was to take home to Isaac.

God audibly spoke to Moses countless times. One that especially stands out in my mind was the time God was so angry at the Israelites for building the golden calf and worshipping it that He told Moses He was going to kill them all and start over— creating a nation of people from Moses rather than Abraham. Let's look at this incident and then talk about it some more...

And the Lord said unto Moses, Go, get thee down; for thy people, which thou broughtest out of the land of Egypt, have corrupted themselves: They have turned aside quickly out of the way which I commanded them: they have made them a molten calf, and have worshipped it, and have sacrificed thereunto, and said, These be thy gods, O Israel, which have brought thee up out of the land of Egypt.

And the Lord said unto Moses, I have seen this people, and, behold, it is a stiffnecked people: Now therefore let me alone, that my wrath may wax hot against them, and that I may consume them: and I will make of thee a great nation. And Moses besought the Lord his God, and said, Lord, why doth thy wrath wax hot against thy people, which thou hast brought forth out of the land of Egypt with great power, and with a mighty hand? Wherefore should the Egyptians speak, and say, For mischief did he bring them out, to slay them in the mountains, and to consume them from the face of the earth?

Turn from thy fierce wrath, and repent of this evil against thy people. Remember Abraham, Isaac, and Israel, thy servants, to whom thou swarest by thine own self, and saidst unto them, I will multiply your seed as the stars of heaven, and all this land that I have spoken of will I give unto your seed, and they shall inherit it for ever. And the Lord repented of the evil which he thought to do unto his people. (Exodus 2:7-14)

Some might say this wasn't actually a prayer, but considering the fact that prayer is conversation between us and God, I'd say it most definitely was. Keeping that in mind, let's take a more in- depth look at what God was *saying* to Moses in this brief encounter:

> God is instructing Moses; telling him to go down to the people.
>
> God is voicing his anger and hurt because Israel was so quick to turn their backs on God.
>
> It would have been or at least tempting (to some degree) for Moses to say, "Go ahead! Wipe them out and make me the new root of your people." But Moses didn't do that. Moses once again proved himself to be the humble servant of God he was.

He reminded God of the promise He made to Abraham and telling God that he was trusting in Him to keep that promise.

God voiced his pleasure with Moses in being so faithful and humble. He then did just what He had promised Abraham and allowed the Israelites to live.

God spoke to Paul when He didn't give Paul what he asked for—to take away whatever chronic ailment (thorn in the flesh) Paul was dealing with.

He wanted Paul to understand that he could be just as effective (if not more so) in the ministry with the ailment as he could without it. God wanted Paul to remember that the work he was doing was *through* him (Paul) *by* God.

FYI: God wants us to know the same.

You listen

The listening part of prayer on our part can be summed up in one word. Obedience.

Jonah didn't listen to God and paid a pretty steep price for his disobedience (Jonah 1). In spite of Jonah's disobedience God still listened to Jonah and gave him another chance.

Ezekiel obeyed God; leading him to have to do some incredibly awkward, humiliating, and 'interesting' things.

Jesus listened to God throughout His life and ministry here on earth, but never so obviously as He did the night He was arrested. Prior to His arrest, Jesus prayed; asking if there was any other way to bring about salvation for you and me. God said no, and Jesus' reply was "Your will be done".

The act of prayer is an act of communication, but it is also what we call a spiritual discipline. The term itself is not found in the Bible, but is one the Church uses to define those things necessary to become more mature and solid in your relationship with God. They are things we need to make part of our character and normal daily lives. You can see by the definition that prayer most certainly falls into that category.

Chapter 2: How to Pray

Jesus out and out told us how we should pray in the Sermon on the Mount (Matthew 5-7). We refer to this instruction in how to pray as the Lord's Prayer. His instruction is primarily what to pray *for* or *about* rather than actually how to pray, so we're going to save that passage of scripture for another chapter. Instead, we're going to look at how to pray as in what our attitude and approach to prayer should be.

Approaching God in Faith

Let's look at a few verses in the Bible on the subject of approaching God in prayer in faith. In doing so we will discover that faith is the key to hearing and receiving God's answers to our prayers.

Therefore I say unto you, What things soever ye desire, when ye pray, believe that ye receive them, and ye shall have them. ~Mark 11:24

This one (and similar verses) are most likely the most misunderstood verse in the Bible. If not, it definitely rates in the top three. Why? Because it is taken out of context, that's why. If you read the verses just prior to this, you will find that Jesus is speaking to the disciples about faith. He tells them that if they have a strong enough faith they can do anything in His name. He then tells them that whatever they ask for they can have, as well. But this is what is called an implied statement. Jesus is implying (not specifically mentioning because the suggestion or understanding is already there) that they wouldn't ask for anything outside the perimeters of one living a faithful, obedient life.

In other words, you wouldn't ask for things that would draw your heart, soul, and mind away from the Father or the Son. You would ask for things (material and otherwise) that would be of physical, emotional, and spiritual benefit to you and to others.

And this is the confidence that we have in him, that, if we ask any thing according to his will, he heareth us: and if we know that he hear us, whatsoever we ask, we know that we have the petitions that we desired of him. 1 John 5:14-15

If ye abide in me, and my words abide in you, ye shall ask what ye will, and it shall be done unto you. ~John 15:7

And all things, whatsoever ye shall ask in prayer, believing, ye shall receive. ~Matthew 21:22

Both of these verses are also on the end of Jesus' comments about the need for faith and being one with Him—heart, soul, and mind.

But let him ask in faith, nothing wavering. For he that wavereth is like a wave of the sea driven with the wind and tossed. For let not that man think that he shall receive any thing of the Lord. A double minded man is unstable in all his ways. ~James 1:6-8

Praying without having faith is like stopping at all the green lights because you don't have faith they will stay green long enough for you to make it through the intersection.

But without faith it is impossible to please him: for he that cometh to God must believe that he is, and that he is a rewarder of them that diligently seek him. ~Hebrews 11:6

This is one of the most beautiful yet telling verses in the Bible. God promises to reward anyone who diligently seeks Him, but reminds us that this is not possible unless we have a faith that is rock-solid. He knows there will be times when we question whether

He is listening because we aren't getting the results we want when we want them. The faith He is talking about here is the faith that never loses sight of the fact that God is real, holy, almighty – and ultimately in control.

Pray Persistently

Pray without ceasing. ~1st Thessalonians 5:17

Call unto me, and I will answer thee, and show thee great and mighty things, which thou knowest not. ~Jeremiah 33:3

Keep asking. Keep talking. Keep listening. God will answer by giving you the promptings of the Holy Spirit, through the works and encouragement of others, and through the events in your life that too many people chalk up to coincidence, happenstance, and fate.

And he spake a parable unto them to this end, that men ought always to pray, and not to faint; Saying, There was in a city a judge, which feared not God, neither regarded man: And there was a widow in that city; and she came unto him, saying, Avenge me of mine adversary. And he would not for a while: but afterward he said within himself, Though I fear not God, nor regard man; yet because this widow troubleth me, I will avenge her, lest by her continual coming she weary me. And the Lord said, Hear what the unjust judge saith. And shall not God avenge his own elect, which cry day and night unto him, though he bear long with them? I tell you that he will avenge them speedily. Nevertheless when the Son of man cometh, shall he find faith on the earth? ~Luke 18:1-18

Jesus' parable is a reminder that God often wants or needs to know how serious or determined we are for what we pray for. Are we genuinely ready for whatever? Are we resolved to handle His answer?

Pray in Agreement with God

Delight thyself also in the Lord: and he shall give thee the desires of thine heart. ~Psalm 37:4

When we are living obediently and faithfully to God, He will give us the desires of our heart because the first desire of our heart will be to do God's will and those that follow will be in line with what God created us to do and be.

Confess your faults one to another, and pray one for another, that ye may be healed. The effectual fervent prayer of a righteous man availeth much. ~James 5:16

For if ye forgive men their trespasses, your heavenly Father will also forgive you: But if ye forgive not men their trespasses, neither will your Father forgive your trespasses. ~Matthew 6:14-15

God cannot and will not answer the prayers of those who refuse to confess their sins to Him or those who refuse to forgive those who have sinned against them.

If my people, which are called by my name, shall humble themselves, and pray, and seek my face, and turn from their wicked ways; then will I hear from heaven, and will forgive their sin, and will heal their land. ~2nd Chronicles 7:14

We must be willing to humble ourselves to the authority and sovereignty of God. We must acknowledge God as the giver of all *because it is all His to give.*

PrayExpectingAnswers

My voice shalt thou hear in the morning, O Lord; in the morning will I direct my prayer unto thee, and will look up. ~Psalm 5:3

David looked up because he knew God was going to answer him. He just knew. I love that because it just shows how sure David was of his God. We should be just as sure today.

Be careful for nothing; but in every thing by prayer and supplication with thanksgiving let your requests be made known unto God. And the peace of God, which passeth all understanding, shall keep your hearts and minds through Christ Jesus. ~Philippians 4:6-7 *He shall call upon me, and I will answer him: I will be with him in trouble; I will deliver him, and honour him.* ~Psalm 91:15

The promise of God should be enough to let us know that our prayers will be answered. It is important to remember, though, that answered prayer isn't always answered the way we want or think it should be.

No parent always tells their child yes, so why should God be any different? He is the God of the 'big picture'. He knows what is going to be and what is best for us in the days, weeks, and years ahead.

But they that wait upon the Lord shall renew their strength; they shall mount up with wings as eagles; they shall run, and not be weary; and they shall walk, and not faint. ~Isaiah 40:31

God's timing is always the perfect timing. We need to remember this—to not get tired of waiting and to not refuse the strength and comfort He offers while we wait. We must also be mindful of not refusing to see God's answer to our prayer if it differs from what we think it should be.

If not, hearken unto me: hold thy peace, and I shall teach thee wisdom. ~Job 33:33

This verse from Job reminds us that in order for God to answer our prayers we have to be quiet long enough to hear Him. Job wanted answers but was too busy telling God he wanted them to hear God speaking. But God got Job's attention—just like He will get ours.

In faith, with persistence and expectation and a heart that longs to be right with God—this is the 'recipe' for how to pray.

Chapter 3: Why Pray

We know what Prayer is and How to Pray . . . But Why Pray? Answering the Why is to understand the motivation behind your actions let me start out by asking this, why do you talk to your best friend, your spouse, your employer, or other people around you? Now sometimes you may not want to talk to your spouse, your employer or even your best friend because of whatever issues that are between you or maybe because you know you're in trouble with your employer.

The fact remains, however, despite whatever the circumstances are in our daily life between these individuals we have to communicate and interact with them just about every day. Why should it be any different with your relationship with God – the one that created you and gave you life?

The short answer is it should not be any different, well let me back up, it should be different if you truly know who God is. So that's the question, who is God to you? When you answer this question you're going to be one step closer to answering a very personal question, why pray?

Now sure there are basic reasons why we should all pray but it really boils down to your relationship with God and who God is to you. The more that you read His Word, the more that you spend time with God in prayer, the more that you draw close to Him the more the God will mean to you.

Recently Valentine's Day had just passed, now I'm not a fan of this particular holiday if that's what you want to call it because I feel that you should be showing your love each and every day to the person that you're with. Nevertheless it brings me to a point to help you better understand something here.

For those that are married do you remember falling in love with your spouse? Do you remember what it was like to have that all-consuming desire and love for them? Do you remember how you couldn't wait until you were able to see them again or talk with them again? We need to have a love relationship with Jesus Christ in a similar fashion. Now I am not talking about a romantic love but a passionate love nonetheless that seeks to have a servant's heart and a sincere desire to do God's will.

Interesting enough if we look at couples that have been married for a long period of time often times you will find the spark has died, they may barely see each other because of work, and hardly ever speak except for talking about the necessities of life such as bills and the kids. This is a great example of how most of our prayer lives are with God.

We have to get back that spark – do you remember when you first came to the Lord how passionate and on fire you were to serve Him and to pray and communicate with him?

Brothers and sisters it's time for a revival within each of us and then collectively as we organically come together in the spirit – let's start a resurrection and a revival once again, and let it start right now within each of us. And then you will understand why you need to pray.

Continuing on with the relationship theme, how many marriages end in divorce because of adultery, abuse or neglect? How many of us have a prayer life that is in similar disarray?

If you're not praying to God but you're sitting in front of the television for hours each day or listening to music is this not adultery if you do not make equal time for God? Are you abusing your relationship with God by only coming to Him in prayer when you need or want something? Are you neglecting your relationship with Almighty God potentially because of sin that is crêpe in and now hold you captive?

Let me explain how the pattern works brothers and sisters first it starts with neglect then it leads to abuse and ultimately adultery

or idolatry as the Bible describes it. It's a vicious cycle but one that can be broken with the blood of the lamb, one that can be broken through committing yourself to learning and getting close to God both in His Word and in Prayer.

Why Pray? Well here's some basic answers:

> Because You Love God
> To Keep Your Relationship with God Strong
> Because You love your family, friends, country etc
> Because you want to see God's will done on Earth as it is in heaven
> To Fight Back Against your Spiritual Enemy
> To Walk in the Authority God has Given You

Remember, prayer is a tangible real thing that should not be discarded or put to the side until you have an emergency or crisis. Is that the kind of relationship you want someone to have with you? Learn to have a good relationship with God by talking with Him daily in prayer.

So many of us continue to struggle and have such a poor prayer life because we don't recognize prayer for what it truly is and just how powerful it is. It should not be your last resort — it should be your immediate response to situations, circumstances, and dealing with our spiritual enemy's attacks.

You must learn to see these attacks for what they are and address them accordingly in prayer — taking authority over the enemy in the name of Jesus. How many of us understand and recognize that every single day of our lives we are in a spiritual war and that prayer is essential for living a victorious life in Christ? Now is the time to Pray!

Chapter 4: Making Time to Pray

Making time to pray is one of the biggest complaints and hurdles Christians say they are faced with. I get it—life is hectic. We have all sorts of people and things vying for our time and attention. It only seems practical or reasonable to put the things that are staring us in the face first. But oh, what a mistake that is!

To help put it into perspective, let me ask you the following questions:

> Would you consider eating dinner and going to bed instead of picking your child up from sports practice or piano lessons because you are at home and able to *see* dinner cooking on the stove and your bedroom, but cannot see your child while they are at practice/lessons?

Would you consider not paying your insurance premiums in order to buy new furniture because you can see the furniture but not the benefits of having the insurance?

Would you not call your parents or grandparents to talk with them or check on their well-being if seeing them on a regular basis was not possible? You know, the 'out of sight, out of mind' philosophy?

I am hoping and praying you answered each of these questions with an emphatic NO. Why, then, do you relegate God and prayer to a status of 'bottom of the totem pole' (last place)?

Whether or not you make time to pray shouldn't be the question. The question should be what you have time for *after* you pray. You might have to give up a television show, a few less minutes in the book you are reading, one less round of golf, or take one less class at the gym, but prayer should take precedence over the activities in your life.

How to make time to pray

If your response to the last statement is something resembling denial that you are too busy or that you cannot possibly give up *that,* you seriously need to re-think your priorities. That being said, I don't want you to feel that what you do with your day is of no importance or significance. That is why I want to offer you the following suggestions on how to make time to pray:

Set aside a special time for prayer each day. A time of completely being focused on conversing with God is essential in your relationship with Him. Think about it: you wouldn't appreciate it if your spouse or your children never took the time to focus on talking to you. You would feel slighted and unimportant. You would feel you were in the way and an inconvenient duty rather than a treasured and cherished loved one.

This is exactly how God feels when we fit Him in when we have a minute here and there or if we are in over our heads and need His divine intervention. By taking the time to be solely focused on prayer each day, you will know God so much more intimately; making it possible for you to avoid many of the issues people use to distance themselves from seeking God's face each day.

Pray before all Meals and as a Family

Pray before you drive anywhere and Pray as you are driving: hands on the wheel, eyes on the road, pray for safety, pray for those you meet on the road, pray for the ability to be a witness of God's goodness in all you do and say throughout your day.

Pray while fixing your kids' breakfast or lunch. Pray for their safety, that they will make right choices, and that they will seek to have a personal relationship with God each and every day of their lives.

Pray while taking a walk. Pray for your community, your church, our government and military, and for those you know who have specific needs.

Pray when you first open your eyes each morning. Thank God for the rest you enjoyed, for His amazing grace, for the fact that He is God, and for the precious gift of salvation.

Pray when you lay your head on the pillow at night. When you make conversation and thoughts of God among the last ones you have each night, you can go to sleep with the peace that passes all understanding.

FYI: Often time's people say they feel guilty falling asleep at night in the middle of their prayers. But I will share with you something I read a while back on that very subject: nothing could be sweeter than drifting off to sleep while talking with your creator. What better company could you possibly have?

Again, I know it isn't always easy to push the hustle and bustle of life out of the way, but for anyone who claims Jesus as Savior, it is something you simply must do in order to make your words more than just lip service. Making prayer a priority is also worth it- Always worth it.

To give you a bit of encouragement and inspiration take a few minutes to read through the following Bible verses. I also encourage and challenge you to commit at least two or three of them to memory so that they can serve as your reminders each and every day.

Pray without ceasing. ~1 Thessalonians 5:17

Any time is a good time to pray. Prayer can be a few words spoken out loud or mentally spoken. Prayer can be a cry for help, a shout of praise, a desperate plea, or a heart to heart conversation that lasts as long as it needs to last.

Likewise the Spirit also helpeth our infirmities: for we know not what we should pray for as we ought: but the Spirit itself maketh intercession for us with groanings which cannot be uttered. ~Romans 8:26

I know someone whose prayer is simply this: "LORD, I know You know what is best and that all things work out for Your good, so please just give me the faith, courage, and strength to hold on for the ride."

But thou, when thou prayest, enter into thy closet, and when thou hast shut thy door, pray to thy Father which is in secret; and thy Father which seeth in secret shall reward thee openly. ~Matthew 6:6

This is the time we spend in focused, personal prayer.

What is it then? I will pray with the spirit, and I will pray with the understanding also: I will sing with the spirit, and I will sing with the understanding also. ~1st Corinthians 14:15

Prayers can also be songs, short and simple words of praise, and thank-yous for God's protection, comfort, and active presence in situations.

Praying always with all prayer and supplication in the Spirit, and watching thereunto with all perseverance and supplication for all saints ~Ephesians 6:18

As for me, I will call upon God; and the Lord shall save me. Evening, and morning, and at noon, will I pray, and cry aloud: and he shall hear my voice. ~Psalm 55:16-17

Again...there's never a bad time to pray.

Chapter 5: Praying the Scriptures

What does it mean to 'pray the scriptures'? The best way to explain it is to pray God's will to be done. It sounds simple because it is. It is also something I can show you better than I can tell you.

Praying the scriptures

Praying for a spouse: *And the Lord God said, It is not good that the man should be alone; I will make him an help meet for him. ~Genesis 2:18*

Praying to know God's will for your life: *For I know the thoughts that I think toward you, saith the Lord, thoughts of peace, and not of evil, to give you an expected end. ~Jeremiah 29:11*

Praying to be more God-centered and a kingdom worker: *But seek ye first the kingdom of God, and his righteousness; and all these things shall be added unto you. ~Matthew 6:33*

Prayer of thanks for your wife: *Whoso findeth a wife findeth a good thing, and obtaineth favour of the Lord.* ~Proverbs 18:22

Pray for increased faith to see God's answers to your prayers: *And blessed is she that believed: for there shall be a performance of those things which were told her from the Lord.* ~Luke 1:45

Pray for Godly parenting skills: *And blessed is she that believed: for there shall be a performance of those things which were told her from the Lord.* ~Ephesians 6:4

Pray for a Godly marriage: *Wives, submit yourselves unto your own husbands, as unto the Lord. Husbands, love your wives, even as Christ also loved the church, and gave himself for it;* ~Ephesians 5:22 and 25

Prayers of thanks for God's gift of salvation: *But God commendeth his love toward us, in that, while we were yet sinners, Christ died for us. ~Romans 5:8*

Pray for the ability to treat those who hurt and persecute you: *But I say unto you, Love your enemies, bless them that curse you, do good to them that hate you, and pray for them which despitefully use you, and persecute you. ~Matthew 5:44*

Prayer of thanks for your friends and loved ones: *I thank my God always on your behalf, for the grace of God which is given you by Jesus Christ ~1 Corinthians 1:4*

Pray for the Church to grow: *Pray ye therefore the Lord of the harvest, that he will send forth labourers into his harvest. ~Matthew 9:38*

Pray to know the mind of Christ for your life: *Ye ask, and receive not, because ye ask amiss, that ye may consume it upon your lusts. ~James 4:3*

Pray for your government and the leaders you work and live under: *I exhort therefore, that, first of all, supplications, prayers, intercessions, and giving of thanks, be made for all men; For kings, and for all that are in authority; that we may lead a quiet and peaceable life in all godliness and honesty. For this is good and acceptable in the sight of God our Saviour; Who will have all men to be saved, and to come unto the knowledge of the truth. ~1 Timothy 2:1-4*

Pray for the lost: *Brethren, my heart's desire and prayer to God for Israel is, that they might be saved. ~Romans 10:1*

Hopefully seeing the scriptures paired with the prayer you can pray helps in understanding what it means to 'pray the scripture'. But just in case it doesn't, here are some examples of what it 'looks like'...

Father, thank You for loving me. Thank You for salvation and your unconditional love. Father, I ask that you give me a heart that seeks Your kingdom and Your righteousness in my life. I pray Your will be my first priority in all things because I know when I live my life in this way You will supply all my needs. (Matthew 6:33) In Jesus' name I pray, amen.

Or...

Father, God, You have said that it is not good for man to be alone. That is why I come to you asking for You to send me the someone I can spend my life with. Send me that special someone who I will love and cherish all the days of my life. I pray he/she will be gentle, faithful to You and to me, and that we can work together to raise children who call You LORD. In Jesus' name I pray, amen. (Genesis 2:18)

Why pray the scriptures

Praying the scriptures serves several purposes—all of which are good and serve to help you grow spiritually. Praying the scriptures:

> Keeps you in focus to pray God's will for yourself and for others

Makes you more knowledgeable of the Word

Allows you to 'cover all the bases' of prayer (thanksgiving, confession, praise, intercession, and petition)

Gives you a more God-centered attitude about life in general

How to pray the scriptures

Praying the scriptures is often done while reading the Bible or during those times when your prayers are brief conversations with specific concerns and/or observations are being made. For example...

If you were reading the book of Proverbs in your daily Bible reading/study, you might pray, "LORD, let me cry out for wisdom and knowledge as the writer of Proverbs tells me to so that I will understand what it means to fear and respect You." (Proverbs 2:3 & 5) Or...

When you are moved by the words of the preacher in a worship service, you might pray, "I am not ashamed of the Gospel and I want You to know, God, that I am committed to living and speaking its truth each and every day with bold grace." (Romans 1:16)

Praying the scriptures won't constitute your entire prayer life, but it will definitely enhance its quality and depth.

Chapter 6: Praying for God's Will to be Done

Similar to praying the Scriptures in the previous chapter, praying for God's will be done is closely related. When you are praying the Scriptures you are praying for specific things that may or may not relate directly to you. God may have specific plans just for you and unfortunately many of us don't know or understand what our calling truly is.

While praying for a wife, wisdom, or the ability to love your enemies are all great things to pray for – what if God's desire for you is not to be married or have children, will you still love Him?

See we don't always get what we want and not everything in Scripture applies directly to us personally -attempting to apply such a philosophy to Scripture would be an error.

It's at these crucial times that we literally Pray for God's will to be done on earth as it is in heaven in our lives – in every aspect of our lives. Pray and ask God to open the doors that He would have you walk through and closed the doors tightly that He would not have you walk through.

Remember Praying without believing is like faith without works – one has to accompany the other to be complete and true. Also remember to keep it real with God, do not simply just pay Him lip service – you're literally wasting your breath.

If you're going to pray for God's will to be done on earth as it is in heaven in your life you have to be ready to accept what that means and what comes next. I think many of us lack the necessary courage and faith to walk out God's will for our lives.

Praying for the necessary courage and faith to walk it out would no doubt be a great prayer if you find yourself doubting or fearful – pray against those things immediately and take authority over them in Jesus name.

Embrace Your Special Needs Child, Prayer, and Parenting
Chapter 7: Jesus Example of Prayer

Jesus Example of Prayer in John 17:

These words spake Jesus, and lifted up his eyes to heaven, and said, Father, the hour is come; glorify thy Son, that thy Son also may glorify thee: As thou hast given him power over all flesh, that he should give eternal life to as many as thou hast given him. And this is life eternal, that they might know thee the only true God, and Jesus Christ, whom thou hast sent. I have glorified thee on the earth: I have finished the work which thou gavest me to do. And now, O Father, glorify thou me with thine own self with the glory which I had with thee before the world was. I have manifested thy name unto the men which thou gavest me out of the world: thine they were, and thou gavest them me; and they have kept thy word. Now they have known that all things whatsoever thou hast given me are of thee. For I have given unto them the words which thou gavest me; and they have received them, and have known surely that I came out from thee, and they have believed that thou didst send me. I pray for them: **I pray not for the world**, but for them which thou hast given me; for they are thine. And all mine are thine, and thine are mine; and I am glorified in them.

And now I am no more in the world, but these are in the world, and I come to thee. Holy Father, keep through thine own name those whom thou hast given me, that they may be one, as we are. While I was with them in the world, I kept them in thy name: those that thou gavest me I have kept, and none of them is lost, but the son of perdition; that the scripture might be fulfilled. And now come I to thee; and these things I speak in the world, that they might have my joy fulfilled in themselves.

I have given them thy word; and the world hath hated them, because they are not of the world, even as I am not of the world. I pray not that thou shouldest take them out of the world, **but that thou shouldest keep them from the evil**. They are not of the world, even as I am not of the world. **Sanctify them through thy truth: thy word is truth.** As thou hast sent me into the world, even so have I also sent them into the world. And for their sakes I sanctify myself, that they also might be sanctified through the truth. **Neither pray I for these alone, but for them also which shall believe on me through their word;** That they all may be one; as thou, Father, art in me, and I in thee, that they also may be one in us: that the world may believe that thou hast sent me.

And the glory which thou gavest me I have given them; that they may be one, even as we are one: I in them, and thou in me, that they may be made perfect in one; and that the world may know that thou hast sent me, and hast loved them, as thou hast loved me. Father, I will that they also, whom thou hast given me, be with me where I am; that they may behold my glory, which thou hast given me: for thou lovedst me before the foundation of the world. O righteous Father, the world hath not known thee: but I have known thee, and these have known that thou hast sent me. And I have declared unto them thy name, and will declare it: that the love wherewith thou hast loved me may be in them, and I in them.

This may in fact be Jesus's longest prayer that is recorded in the New Testament, let's look at some key things that stand out in this prayer. First and foremost it's important to recognize that in this particular prayer Jesus does not pray for the world but for those that believe in Him – His disciples and those that would believe because of the disciple's words. Jesus also prays that his father would keep them from evil and sanctify them through God's word.

It's amazing that over 2000 years ago when Christ prayed these words that He was thinking about you and I who believe in Him because of the apostles words written down in the Holy Bible. What an awesome God we serve.

In this prayer we read how Jesus interacts with the father – does your prayer life look like this? How do you pray for the disciples that you should be making? How do you pray for future generations that will believe because of those disciples' words? Are you even making disciples? Are you going about your father's business – will you hear the words well done good and faithful servant? In this prayer Jesus knows He is about to return back to the father and that His time is short, it's almost like He's reviewing a checklist for things that he needed to do while He was on earth.

We, however, do not know when our time on this earth will be completed therefore it is critical to pray with a sense of urgency as if eternity is just around the corner. The more that you study this specific prayer the more you will have insight into the heart of Jesus Christ.

"The Lord's Prayer"

Jesus' words to His disciples in regards to instructing them (and us) how to pray are what we refer to as the Lord's Prayer. The passage of scripture found in Matthew 6 is often recited and memorized as an actual prayer. Quite honestly, however, this is not what it was intended to be. Jesus' intentions weren't for us to recite

His words. His intentions were for us to pattern our prayers according to His outline'.

This might bring up the question of whether or not it is wrong to pray the Lord's Prayer. My answer to that would be no—that it is not *wrong*, but I would add to that by saying it is not really beneficial to do so. I say this because:

> The Lord's Prayer is not *personal* and from the heart— as prayer should be.

Praying the Lord's Prayer might be considered praying the scripture, but unless you make it specific, you are reciting, not praying.

That being said...the Lord's Prayer is a good way to teach yourself or others how to stay focused on praying for and about the things we need to pray for. So let's take a look at the Lord's Prayer; taking it apart line by line to see what Jesus is wanting us to learn from His model prayer.

After this manner therefore pray ye: Our Father which art in heaven, Hallowed be thy name. Thy kingdom come, Thy will be done in earth, as it is in heaven. Give us this day our daily bread. And forgive us our debts, as we forgive our debtors. And lead us not into temptation, but deliver us from evil: For thine is the kingdom, and the power, and the glory, forever. Amen. ~Matthew 6:9-13

Our Father in heaven, hallowed be thy name:

Recognizing God for who He is should always be first in your daily prayer sessions. When you recognize God you are naturally humbled. Doing so also prepares your heart for speaking, listening, and obeying because it affirms your faith and belief in God's holiness.

God isn't picky when it comes to what you say to 'hallow His name'. A simple thank-you for being God will do, but it isn't difficult to come up with a whole lot more than that. You can also praise God for His holiness by recognizing any of the many attributes of His character. For example, some of the character traits the Bible attributes to God include:

Personally interested—God is personally interested in every little detail of your life. He has the hairs on your head numbered as well as the days of your life. He has a lot invested in you and is constantly watching and waiting for a return on that investment.

Creator of all—all of creation is God's to do with as He pleases. To praise God for the intricate workings of nature should be as natural as breathing.

Vine pruner—God prunes and shapes our lives so that we can live out our purpose. Discipline is a part of growing and maturing. To expect otherwise is prideful and honestly, quite delusional. Who are we to think God shouldn't correct us?

When done correctly, discipline is an excellent teacher as well as serving to hone our skills and character. FYI: God always 'does discipline' the right way.

Truth—God's Word is true and unchanging and He is always good for the many promises He has made.

Savior—God's mercy and unconditional love are the only reason we have salvation from sin that offers the opportunity to spend eternity with Him.

Eternal—God is forever and nothing is going to change that.

Forgiving—when we sincerely ask forgiveness God is always ready, willing, and able to forgive. This is the greatest attribute of all.

Thy kingdom come, Thy will be done in earth, as it is in heaven. I am quite certain that most people reciting these words don't truly understand what it is they are saying or asking for. I am also equally certain they don't realize the responsibility they are signing on for when they say these words. I don't say this to be critical or to sound as if I am on a higher level of spirituality. I am simply trying to help each of us come to a more intimate and genuine level of communication with God. So let's take a closer look at this phrase and what it really means...

Thy kingdom come. Jesus is really saying two things here.

He is saying we should be praying with anticipation for God to sound the trumpet for the second coming of Christ. That's pretty straightforward and easy to understand. But it is also something many people *say* they look forward to, but... To ask God to come soon should come from a heart that truly looks forward with assurance and hope for eternity in heaven.

Jesus is also talking about the growth of the Kingdom of God here on earth. In many of Jesus' parables He says "..the kingdom of God..." or "...the kingdom of heaven...".

In both instances Jesus is referring to you and me here as in the body of saved believers. He is instructing us to pray for the development of the Kingdom of God within us and for the Kingdom to grow and spread across the world so that as many as possible might come to know Jesus as Savior. This is definitely something we should be praying for.

Now for our role in this: in praying for the growth and spreading of the Kingdom of God, we are saying we will do our part to make that happen.

We are basically saying, "Bring on the Great Commission! I'm ready to get down to the business of making Disciples!"

But are you? Am I? Are we really willing to help God's kingdom increase here on earth? If so, what are we actively doing to try to make that happen in our own little corner of the world?

Thy will be done in earth, as it is in heaven. This is simply Jesus' way of emphasizing what He had just said—to remind us that God's kingdom wasn't just some far-off place. Jesus was reminding us that we have a job to do here on earth and that job is to be God's living, breathing, and active representatives of His Kingdom. We are to be about the business of God each and every day of our lives. This sentence in the model prayer is to remind us that we shouldn't be shy or scared to ask God for a daily supply of courage, strength, wisdom, compassion, discernment, and love to be who and what we are supposed to be.

Give us this day our daily bread. We are to ask God for the things we need—bread and everything else.

Sometimes we are so naïve. Or maybe it's pride. Either way we are often blind to the fact that everything we have belongs to God. He gives us the ability to earn a salary from which we buy the things we enjoy and have to have, but it all goes back to the fact that *He gives us the ability.*

Asking God to provide our needs and the desires of our heart humbles us to recognize our inability to make due on our own and the fact that these things are God's to give as He pleases. We are expressing our need for God's care and provision.

And forgive us our debts, as we forgive our debtors. The words 'debt' and 'debtors' in the original Greek means 'that which is due'. Using this direct translation of the word, let's look at what Jesus is saying:

Forgive us for not giving You that which is due in the same way we forgive those who don't give us that which is due us.

I see a bit of Jesus' irony coming out here. He is instructing us to ask God for the same measure of forgiveness we extend to others. Ouch!

By instructing us in this way, Jesus is reminding us of three things:

> Jesus is reminding us of our need for grace—that none of us is any more deserving of God's favor than the person next to us.

Jesus is reminding us that we are all sinners and that in God's eyes no sin is greater than another.

> Jesus is reminding us of what He had just said about loving our enemies, not holding grudges, and going the extra mile (Matthew 5).

Immediately following the model for prayer, Jesus goes on to say this:

For if ye forgive men their trespasses, your heavenly Father will also forgive you: But if ye forgive not men their trespasses, neither will your Father forgive your trespasses. ~Matthew 6:14-15

The word 'trespasses' in the Greek is translated 'to step over' or 'sin'. I'm not sure why He used the word 'trespass' here and the word 'debtor' in giving us the model prayer, but it is obvious He is tying the two together. He knows that an unforgiving heart cannot be in alignment with doing the will of God. That is why He instructed us to pray this for ourselves each and every day.

And lead us not into temptation, but deliver us from evil...

When I read this I think of the old hymn, "I Need Thee Every Hour". Part of it goes like this:

I need Thee every hour; stay close and nearby. Temptations lose their power when You are close by. I need Thee, Oh, I need Thee. Every hour I need Thee. Oh, bless me now my Savior, I come to Thee.

The Bible tells us in no uncertain terms that neither God nor Jesus tempts us—that temptation comes from the devil. He plants it like seeds in our hearts and minds. He puts it before us in cunning disguises, but it is always from him. The devil is also very persuasive in his ability to tempt us. Jesus knows that. He also knows that we need to stay in prayer if we are going to walk in victory against the devil and his minions.

For thine is the kingdom, and the power, and the glory, forever. Amen. The ending of our prayer should be to bring it full-circle; putting the focus back on God. Ending our prayer time by giving God the glory and recognition he deserves is only fitting. Ending our prayers this way also serves as just one more reminder of the fact that we are reliant on and hopeful in God.

There are a number of things people do to assist them in establishing a consistent prayer life. We're going to look at several of them in the next chapter, but I want to close this section of the book by saying that when it comes to the 'mechanics' of prayer, Jesus' model prayer is much more than an idea or suggestion. It is an instruction...command, even...from Jesus the Savior and only Son of God

Chapter 8: Learning to be a Prayer Warrior

A prayer warrior—sounds a little intimidating, doesn't it? Don't worry, though. It's not. A prayer warrior is merely a term used to describe someone who is vigilant and ceaseless in their prayers. A prayer warrior is someone who knows and counts on the power of prayer to bring about change and blessing in their life and the lives of others. A Prayer Warrior is someone who understands there is a Spiritual War going on all the time. They intercede for themselves and others by binding, rebuking, and taking authority over the enemy through faith and prayer. A prayer warrior is someone who understands the power of prayer and the authority Christ has given us and operates in faith and courage to do battle against spiritual forces of darkness.

I mentioned at the conclusion of a previous chapter that there are several methods people use to help them establish a strong and consistent prayer life. We're going to look at a few of them now in an effort to help you do the same.

Pray without ceasing

You have seen this verse sprinkled throughout the pages of this book and here it is again: *Pray without ceasing. ~1st Thessalonians 5:17* Your mom always told you that practice makes perfect when it came time to practice your music lessons, or learn your multiplication facts. Well, the same holds true for the discipline of prayer. Practice makes perfect. The more you pray the more you will want to pray and the more you want to pray the more reliant you will become on God. And that, my friend, is about as perfect as it gets this side of heaven.

ACTS Acronym

Adoration: Giving God the glory, praise and honor due Him.

Praising God for creation and for His forever-ness.

> *Who being the brightness of his glory, and the express image of his person, and upholding all things by the word of his power, when he had by himself purged our sins, sat down on the right hand of the Majesty on high: ~Hebrews 1:3*

> *And every creature which is in heaven, and on the earth, and under the earth, and such as are in the sea, and all that are in them, heard I saying, Blessing, and honour, and glory, and power, be unto him that sitteth upon the throne, and unto the Lamb for ever and ever. ~Revelation 5:13*

And thou shalt love the Lord thy God with all thy heart, and with all thy soul, and with all thy mind, and with all thy strength: this is the first commandment. ~Mark 12:30

Praise ye the Lord. Praise God in his sanctuary: praise him in the firmament of his power. Praise him for his mighty acts: praise him according to his excellent greatness. Praise him with the sound of the trumpet: praise him with the psaltery and harp. Praise him with the timbrel and dance: praise him with stringed instruments and organs. Praise him upon the loud cymbals: praise him upon the high sounding cymbals. Let every thing that hath breath praise the Lord. Praise ye the Lord. ~Psalm 150

Confession: Confessing your sins to God specifically, humbly, and with a heart of true repentance.

> *If we confess our sins, he is faithful and just to forgive us our sins, and to cleanse us from all unrighteousness. ~1st John 1:9*

> *He that covereth his sins shall not prosper: but whoso confesseth and forsaketh them shall have mercy. ~Proverbs 28:13*

> *Submit yourselves therefore to God. Resist the devil, and he will flee from you. Draw nigh to God, and he will draw nigh to you. Cleanse your hands, ye sinners; and purify your hearts, ye double minded. Be afflicted, and mourn, and weep: let your laughter be turned to mourning, and your joy to heaviness. Humble yourselves in the sight of the Lord, and he shall lift you up. ~James 4:7-10*

Have mercy upon me, O God, according to thy lovingkindness: according unto the multitude of thy tender mercies blot out my transgressions. Wash me throughly from mine iniquity, and cleanse me from my sin. For I acknowledge my transgressions: and my sin is ever before me. ~Psalm 51:1-3

Thanksgiving: Give thanks to God for His blessings, His love, His mercy, His gift of salvation, and for the hope of heaven.

Giving thanks always for all things unto God and the Father in the name of our Lord Jesus Christ; ~Ephesians 5:20

O give thanks unto the God of heaven: for his mercy endureth for ever. ~Psalm 136:26

> *Bless the Lord, O my soul, and forget not all his benefits...*
> *~Psalm 103:2*

> *Enter into his gates with thanksgiving, and into his courts with praise: be thankful unto him, and bless his name.*
> *~Psalm 100:4*

Supplication: Praying on behalf of others and asking for the things we need and desire is definitely a part of prayer. Remember: prayer is communicating with God for the purpose of developing a deeper relationship with Him. That cannot happen if we aren't honest with God and if we don't open ourselves up completely to Him.

> *And this is the confidence that we have in him, that, if we ask any thing according to his will, he heareth us...*
> *~1st John 5:14*

Ye ask, and receive not, because ye ask amiss, that ye may consume it upon your lusts. ~James 4:3

But let him ask in faith, nothing wavering. For he that wavereth is like a wave of the sea driven with the wind and tossed. For let not that man think that he shall receive any thing of the Lord. A double minded man is unstable in all his ways. ~James 1:6-8

My help cometh from the Lord, which made heaven and earth. ~Psalm 121:2

Come unto me, all ye that labour and are heavy laden, and I will give you rest. ~Matthew 11:28

And the Lord turned the captivity of Job, when he prayed for his friends: also the Lord gave Job twice as much as he had before. ~Job 42:10

PRAY Acronym

The PRAY acronym is another often-used method of developing good prayer habits. As you can see, it is quite similar to the ACTS acronym, but then why wouldn't it be? They all follow the model prayer (the LORD's prayer) in Matthew 6.

There is, however, one aspect of the PRAY acronym I think needs to be highlighted. It is the Y, which reminds us to yield to God's purpose for our lives. So while I won't take the time to repeat every scripture used above for the ACTS acronym, I will insert a few of them in the appropriate place then focus on some that deal with yielding to God's will.

Praise: Giving God the glory, praise and honor due Him.

Praising God for creation and for His forever-ness.

> *Who being the brightness of his glory, and the express image of his person, and upholding all things by the word of his power, when he had by himself purged our sins, sat down on the right hand of the Majesty on high: ~Hebrews 1:3*

And every creature which is in heaven, and on the earth, and under the earth, and such as are in the sea, and all that are in them, heard I saying, Blessing, and honour, and glory, and power, be unto him that sitteth upon the throne, and unto the Lamb for ever and ever.
~Revelation 5:13

Repent: To repent means to change your ways. It is a reversing of yourself from living a sinful lifestyle to a Godly lifestyle.

And the times of this ignorance God winked at; but now commandeth all men every where to repent... Acts 17:30

Know ye not that the unrighteous shall not inherit the kingdom of God? Be not deceived: neither fornicators, nor idolaters, nor adulterers, nor effeminate, nor abusers of themselves with mankind, nor thieves, nor covetous, nor drunkards, nor revilers, nor extortioners, shall inherit the kingdom of God. ~1 Corinthians 6:9-10

Then Peter said unto them, Repent, and be baptized every one of you in the name of Jesus Christ for the remission of sins, and ye shall receive the gift of the Holy Ghost. ~Acts 2:38

And be not conformed to this world: but be ye transformed by the renewing of your mind, that ye may prove what is that good, and acceptable, and perfect, will of God.
~Romans 12:2

And fear not them which kill the body, but are not able to kill the soul: but rather fear him which is able to destroy both soul and body in hell. ~Matthew 10:28

Ask: Asking God for the desires of your heart, for the needs you have in your life, and for the provision and safety for others all comes under this 'category'.

Ye ask, and receive not, because ye ask amiss, that ye may consume it upon your lusts. ~James 4:3

But let him ask in faith, nothing wavering. For he that wavereth is like a wave of the sea driven with the wind and tossed. For let not that man think that he shall receive any thing of the Lord. A double minded man is unstable in all his ways. ~James 1:6-8

My help cometh from the Lord, which made heaven and earth. ~Psalm 121:2

Come unto me, all ye that labour and are heavy laden, and I will give you rest. ~Matthew 11:28

Yield: To yield is to give in—to allow God to have His way in your life. Yielding is submission and obedience. Yielding is also living by faith.

For God so loved the world, that he gave his only begotten Son, that whosoever believeth in him should not perish, but have everlasting life. ~John 3:16

What? know ye not that your body is the temple of the Holy Ghost which is in you, which ye have of God, and ye are not your own? ~1st Corinthians 6:19

Trust in the Lord with all thine heart; and lean not unto thine own understanding. In all thy ways acknowledge him, and he shall direct thy paths. Be not wise in thine own eyes: fear the Lord, and depart from evil. ~Proverbs 3:5-7

But be ye doers of the word, and not hearers only, deceiving your own selves. For if any be a hearer of the word, and not a doer, he is like unto a man beholding his natural face in a glass:

For he beholdeth himself, and goeth his way, and straightway forgetteth what manner of man he was. But whoso looketh into the perfect law of liberty, and continueth therein, he being not a forgetful hearer, but a doer of the work, this man shall be blessed in his deed. ~James 1:22-25

Be ye therefore followers of God, as dear children. ~Ephesians 5:1

For if we sin wilfully after that we have received the knowledge of the truth, there remaineth no more sacrifice for sins, But a certain fearful looking for of judgment and fiery indignation, which shall devour the adversaries. ~Hebrews 10:26-27

God is a Spirit: and they that worship him must worship him in spirit and in truth. ~John 4:24

I'll say it again: a prayer warrior is someone who understands, believes in, and depends on the power of prayer. Be a prayer warrior!

Chapter 9: Praying for Healing

Praying for the healing of self and others is something many of us have difficulty in wrapping our heads and hearts around. We pray believing God will hear us. We pray believing God will give us what we ask for because that is what scripture tells us. We pray, yet much of the time our prayers are not answered in the way we think they should be. Our loved one dies. An innocent child is taken from the loving arms of their parents. Soldiers don't come home.

So what's the matter? Are we praying wrong? Is the Bible lying? The answers to those questions are as follows:

We may or may not be praying 'wrong'. While it is never wrong to ask God to heal someone so that we can continue to enjoy loving them here on earth or so that their families can remain intact, our first prayer should always be for God's will to be done because His will is always perfect and right. Secondly we can pray for those we wish to pray for, but along with those prayers we should ask God for the strength and wisdom necessary to accept His answer.

Right now a young family in the Midwest is praying earnestly for their infant son. He has a somewhat rare disease that has robbed him of his ability to swallow on his own, to sit or stand, and of the ability for his lungs to expel fluid. This little guy has to spend most of his time hooked to one machine or another. He will likely not reach his second birthday. His parents, grandparents, and countless friends, family, and other prayer warriors are praying for baby Logan and his family.

They are praying for miraculous healing. But they are also praying for strength, courage, and wisdom to give him the best of their love for whatever time God gives them together.

No, the Bible is not lying. The Bible tells us that whatever we ask for in God's will it will be done. Yet we have to remember God's will first - Always first.

Keeping that in mind, let's take a look at some of the scriptures dealing with prayers for healing. As you read them, think about how you can be more in tune to God's will and prayers for His children.

Most of all remember this: Healing in its best and truest form is to be with God the Father for all eternity. Not to sound morbid or anything but for those who are saved but dealing with terminal illness, healing is often physical death.

> *Is any among you afflicted? let him pray. Is any merry? let him sing psalms. Is any sick among you? let him call for the elders of the church; and let them pray over him, anointing him with oil in the name of the Lord: And the prayer of faith shall save the sick, and the Lord shall raise him up; and if he have committed sins, they shall be forgiven him. Confess your faults one to another, and pray one for another, that ye may be healed. The effectual fervent prayer of a righteous man availeth much. ~James 5:13-16*

And we know that all things work together for good to them that love God, to them who are the called according to his purpose. ~Romans 8:28

Beloved, I wish above all things that thou mayest prosper and be in health, even as thy soul prospereth. ~3rd John 1:2

Who his own self bare our sins in his own body on the tree, that we, being dead to sins, should live unto righteousness: by whose stripes ye were healed. ~1st Peter 2:24

As I mentioned before when are prayers don't get answered, especially prayers for love ones healing it can cause confusion and doubt in your faith and sometimes even in God. Yet this is a snare of the devil to keep you locked in bondage – learn to break free from the oppression of the devil by walking in faith, encourage, and in the word of God. One way to break free from this oppression in bondage is to develop a checklist of sorts.

Consider the following is a short checklist:

Is there sin in my life preventing my prayers from being answered

Do I know for certain what I'm praying is God's will? – If not then pray that God's will would be done on earth as it is in heaven in the situation.

I'm I being targeted by workers of darkness such as witches, Satanist, and others who practice the dark arts?

Have I cleansed myself from all generational curses or familiar spirits?

Is my relationship with God where it needs to be?

Have I prayed over my house or place of continual prayer?

Is there an open door that I or my family members have inadvertently opened to enable the spiritual forces of darkness to hinder my prayer life?

Are there things in my home that are spiritually charged that are affecting my prayer life?

Have I done my due diligence, and through the Spirit of God attempted to research and rightly divide the Word of God as it pertains to the specific situation?

These are just a few questions to ask yourself when you're prayers are not being answered. Sometimes it's also critical to fast and pray — remember it's a real war and it's here every day.

Chapter 10: Praying as a Means of Spiritual Warfare

Spiritual Warfare sounds even scarier and more intimidating than the term 'Prayer Warrior'. That's because it can actually be a very scary thing if you don't know what you're doing or who you are in Christ Jesus. Learn from the clear example below in the Word of God not to try this unless you know who you are in Christ.

Acts 19:11-17
Now God worked unusual miracles by the hands of Paul, so that even handkerchiefs or aprons were brought from his body to the sick, and the diseases left them and the evil spirits went out of them. Then some of the itinerant Jewish exorcists took it upon themselves to call the name of the Lord Jesus over those who had evil spirits, saying, "We exorcise you by the Jesus whom Paul preaches." Also there were seven sons of Sceva, a Jewish chief priest, who did so. And the evil spirit answered and said, "Jesus I know, and Paul I know; <u>but who are you</u>?"

Then the man in whom the evil spirit was leaped on them, over powered them, and prevailed against them, so that they fled out of that house naked and wounded. This became known both to all Jews and Greeks dwelling in Ephesus; and fear fell on them all, and the name of the Lord Jesus was magnified.

Now I'm not trying to scare you here but you have to understand there is a real war going on between the Kingdom of God and the kingdom of the devil. This is a spiritual war with earthly consequences. Fallen Angels, demons, and demonic possession are all very real things and is not something that the novice should get into with little to no training.

One of the best men of God in our age to learn from is Russ Dizdar. His website is www.shatterthedarkness.com for those interested in learning more about his ministry.

We don't need to be scared of the devil but mindful of his ways and unrelenting attacks on our hearts, souls, minds, and bodies.

Be sober, be vigilant; because your adversary the devil walks about like a roaring lion, seeking whom he may devour. Resist him, steadfast in the faith, knowing that the same sufferings are experienced by your brotherhood in the world - 1 Peter 5:8-9

lest Satan should take advantage of us; for we are not ignorant of his devices - 2 Cor. 2:11

Therefore submit to God. Resist the devil and he will flee from you. – James 4:7

We don't need to be afraid of what the devil can do to us, we have been given authority over him and all his evil minions. We don't need to even be afraid of being separated from God somehow either here on earth or for all eternity. Let's let the Scriptures speak for themselves, below you can see that nothing can separate us from the love of God in Christ Jesus in addition to Christ giving us all authority to trample on serpents and scorpions and over all the power of the enemy – did you see the word all. That sounds pretty absolute to me. The main thing that we need to realize here is what manner of spirit we are of – 2 Tim 1:7 makes it very clear that God has not given us a spirit of fear, but of power, and of love, and of a sound mind.

For I am persuaded that neither death nor life, nor angels nor principalities nor powers, nor things present nor things to come, nor height nor depth, nor any other created thing, shall be able to separate us from the love of God which is in Christ Jesus our Lord - Rom. 8:38-39

You are of God, little children, and have overcome them, because He who is in you is greater than he who is in the world -1 John 4:4

Then the seventy returned with joy, saying, "Lord, even the demons are subject to us in Your name." And He said to them, "I saw Satan fall like lightning from heaven. Behold, I give you the authority to trample on serpents and scorpions, and over all the power of the enemy, and nothing shall by any means hurt you. Nevertheless do not rejoice in this, that the spirits are subject to you, but rather rejoice because your names are written in heaven - Luke 10:17-20

For God has not given us a spirit of fear, but of power and of love and of a sound mind 2 Tim 1:7

There is no fear in love; but perfect love casts out fear, because fear involves torment. But he who fears has not been made perfect in love. 1 John 4:18

Spiritual warfare is very real. Look around you - the social unrest, the violence in our schools and in our streets, the persecution of Christians around the world (including here in the US), and the demoralizing of our society screams spiritual attacks from the devil and his minions.

The devil is on the move and making great strides because he knows his time is short - *[7] And war broke out in heaven: Michael and his angels fought with the dragon; and the dragon and his angels fought, [8] but they did not prevail, nor was a place found for them in heaven any longer.*

[9] So the great dragon was cast out, that serpent of old, called the Devil and Satan, who deceives the whole world; he was cast to the earth, and his angels were cast out with him. [10] Then I heard a loud voice saying in heaven, "Now salvation, and strength, and the kingdom of our God, and the power of His Christ have come, for the accuser of our brethren, who accused them before our God day and night, has been cast down.

11 And they overcame him by the blood of the Lamb and by the word of their testimony, and they did not love their lives to the death.
12 Therefore rejoice, O heavens, and you who dwell in them! **Woe to the inhabitants of the earth and the sea! For the devil has come down to you, having great wrath, because he knows that he has a short time."** *Rev. 12:7-12*

But know this: God has already won, He is Victorious. He has already Won the War and those who are in Christ have the Victory – IF They Claim It and Walk in It

Let these verses equip you for the battles to come:

For we wrestle not against flesh and blood, but against principalities, against powers, against the rulers of the darkness of this world, against spiritual wickedness in high places.
~Ephesians 6:12

Above all, taking the shield of faith, wherewith ye shall be able to quench all the fiery darts of the wicked. ~Ephesians 6:16

Be sober, be vigilant; because your adversary the devil, as a roaring lion, walketh about, seeking whom he may devour
~1st Peter 5:8

Submit yourselves therefore to God. Resist the devil, and he will flee from you. ~James 4:7

For whatsoever is born of God overcometh the world: and this is the victory that overcometh the world, even our faith. Who is he that overcometh the world, but he that believeth that Jesus is the Son of God?
~1st John 5:4-5

No weapon that is formed against thee shall prosper; and every tongue that shall rise against thee in judgment thou shalt condemn. This is the heritage of the servants of the Lord, and their righteousness is of me, saith the Lord.
~Isaiah 54:17

The Scriptures above are clear and to the point – we have the authority, we have the victory, we have everything we need to defeat the devil and everything he throws at us if we have the courage and the faith to believe God's Word enough to take action in our daily lives. Will you boldly walk out your faith today?

Praying for your enemies

Let's briefly discuss praying for your enemies. There are several reasons that if you're a follower of Jesus Christ should pray for your enemies. First and foremost we have to guard against hatred and resentment building up within our spirit. Hatred and resentment is like a spiritual cancer that infects our spirit separating us from completing God's perfect will for our life.

There is a fundamental Christian principle that Christ taught us and that is to be forgiven we have to forgive others – it's just that simple.

A lot of times when we do not forgive someone, in all reality it's only affecting us - the other person probably has no clue of the entirety of your feelings.

Let's once again look to the Scripture for clarification:

Matt.5:43-47

[43] "You have heard that it was said, 'You shall love your neighbor and hate your enemy.' [44] But I say to you, love your enemies, bless those who curse you, do good to those who hate you, and pray for those who spitefully use you and persecute you, [45] that you may be sons of your Father in heaven; for He makes His sun rise on the evil and on the good, and sends rain on the just and on the unjust. [46] For if you love those who love you,

what reward have you? Do not even the tax collectors do the same? [47] And if you greet your brethren only, what do you do more than others? Do not even the tax collectors do so? [48] Therefore you shall be perfect, just as your Father in heaven is perfect.

Rom. 12:9-21

Let love be without hypocrisy. Abhor what is evil. Cling to what is good. Be kindly affectionate to one another with brotherly love, in honor giving preference to one another; not lagging in diligence, fervent in spirit, serving the Lord; rejoicing in hope, patient in tribulation, continuing steadfastly in prayer; distributing to the needs of the saints, given to hospitality. Bless those who persecute you; bless and do not curse. Rejoice with those who rejoice, and weep with those who weep. Be of the same mind toward one another. Do not set your mind on high things, but associate with the humble. Do not be wise in your own opinion.

Repay no one evil for evil. Have regard for good things in the sight of all men. If it is possible, as much as depends on you, live peaceably with all men. Beloved, do not avenge yourselves, but rather give place to wrath; for it is written, "Vengeance is Mine, I will repay," says the Lord. Therefore "If your enemy is hungry, feed him; If he is thirsty, give him a drink; For in so doing you will heap coals of fire on his head." Do not be overcome by evil, but overcome evil with good.

Releasing this type of hatred, resentment, and unforgiveness cleanses your spirit as you repent of these things and enables you to draw closer to God. Now this is not to say that there isn't a time and a place for righteous anger. The Bible declares that you can be angry and not sin but you have to be led by the Word of God and His Holy Spirit

Chapter 11: Developing Your Prayer List

What is a prayer list?

The simple definition of a prayer list according to yours truly is simply a list of items that you feel compelled to pray for – normally the items on this list are prayed for when I consistent basis every day until God puts it on your heart to move on to something else. For example praying for the salvation of a loved one by their specific name, or if a relative is dealing with a sickness or illness.

Getting Serious!

Developing a prayer list could potentially be one sign that you're starting to take prayer more serious.

It's an indication that you understand the power and the value of praying consistently each and every day to affect change in the dynamics you're dealing with. I found this to be true in my case. Sure I prayed as the Spirit led, or when there was a need but slowly the Holy Spirit put within my heart a burden for the salvation of my mother and other people around me and it was at this point that I started writing down things to pray for and putting it up where I could see it continually. See I'm a visual person and a lot of times if I don't see it I will forget it – I'm sure a lot of you can relate to this, especially with how hectic life can be.

Therefore, I cannot stress strongly enough that

once you've created a prayer list that you put it up somewhere in which you will continually see it such as a home office. Oh – make sure you either write it large enough to see it or type it in a font that's large enough for you to see it from a distance.

The bottom line is just to keep it in front of you and in your mind. Don't let prayers go one prayed because of lack of discipline and spiritual laziness. To be a strong Christian prayer warrior requires discipline, vigilance, and the warrior spirit that the Lord himself will mold you into.

The Why

The Why is straightforward here. We all forget things, that's just a reality of life, don't beat yourself up about it just keep it moving ever adapting to changes and situations that the devil attempts to throw at you. As you continue to develop into a prayer warrior your intensity, passion, and desire to serve the living God will increase to the point where you will continually walk victorious – remember you are Christ's ambassadors, the King of Kings and the Lord of lords.

An Example of My Prayer List

In this section I want to share with you my personal prayer list. This is my general list of things that I pray for or about on a consistent basis. Please note the order in which I list them as there is a systematic order in which I pray from the first thing to the last thing (normally).

They are as follows:

> Giving Thanks – showing my appreciation for all that God is doing, has done, and will do
>
> Repentance - this is something I pray as needed
>
> Protection - pleading the blood of Jesus over me and my family and those around us
>
> Salvation - for my family members, neighbors, and specific people my life
>
> Healing - if there is a specific medical need, but at times I pray that salvation and healing walk hand-in-hand
>
> Revival - that God would stir the hearts and minds of his people
>
> Brothers and Sisters in Christ - for protection, healing, leading, for God's perfect will to be done in their lives

For Leadership in Government - this includes America and Israel

Workers for the harvest -this is praying the Scriptures - for God to send workers

Prayer Warriors -for God to raise up Prayer Warriors

Those Most Vulnerable in Our Society - in this area I pray for the elderly, the sick and affirmed, the homeless and hungry, those in foster care, those still within their mother's womb, and for the children worldwide to be protected. In this section I start to really get into spiritual warfare. I pray against the spiritual forces behind pedophile rings, Satanic networks, human trafficking networks, sex trafficking networks.

I pray that the Lord would send His angels – yes is holy and righteous Angels to protect every single person in our society without a voice who may be being abused, tortured, molested, or maybe they have been kidnapped, and may soon be sacrificed to the enemy.

Then ask God specifically to help us and the systematic murder of the children that are still yet in her mother's womb – this Holocaust, this bloodshed has to come to an end if our nation has any chance for redemption. Because understand this this bloodshed is literally part of sacrifices to the devil. Many people don't understand that blood is a currency in the amount of innocent blood that has been shed is overwhelming – help me pray against this brothers and sisters. Through prayer we can shine God's light into the darkness was focus our efforts together in prayer and shine God's light into the darkness to expose this evil and abolish it from our land.

> Against the Enemy - after I've begun to pray for those most vulnerable in our society and against the demonic forces that seek to destroy them I then shift gears and specifically go after the spiritual enemy even more.

Chapter 12: When It Seems God Doesn't Hear Your Prayers

When God Doesn't Answer Prayers?

We've touched on this already to some degree but let's examine some times in Scripture were men of "Faith" don't have their prayers answered or answered immediately.

> Daniel - Prince of Persia holding him up
>
> The Disciples of Jesus – Faithless, Perversion, Jesus said, "Because of your unbelief"
>
> Job - A perfect example of following God faithfully and having sudden destruction fall upon you similar to the way we may pray but not necessarily see an answer to our prayers. God allowed Satan to attack Job and his family – but what you see here is that whatever is happening God is still in charge. Satan had to come and get God's permission to do anything to Job. So even

though times may seem dark you are still in the palm of his hand if you faithfully abide in Christ.

The question you should ask yourself is this – Are you just honoring God with your mouth but your heart is far from Him?

This people draweth nigh unto me with their mouth, and honoureth me with their lips; but their heart is far from me. Matt. 15:8

Dan. 10:12-13

^{12} Then said he unto me, Fear not, Daniel: for from the first day that thou didst set thine heart to understand, and to chasten thyself before thy God, thy words were heard, and I am come for thy words. ^{13} But the prince of the kingdom of Persia withstood me one and twenty days: but, lo, Michael, one of the chief princes, came to help me; and I remained there with the kings of Persia.

Matt. 17:15-21

¹⁵ Lord, have mercy on my son: for he is lunatick, and sore vexed: for often times he falleth into the fire, and often into the water. ¹⁶ And I brought him to thy disciples, and they could not cure him.

¹⁷ Then Jesus answered and said, O faithless and perverse generation, how long shall I be with you? how long shall I suffer you? bring him hither to me. ¹⁸ And Jesus rebuked the devil; and he departed out of him: and the child was cured from that very hour. ¹⁹ Then came the disciples to Jesus apart, and said, Why could not we cast him out? ²⁰ And Jesus said unto them, Because of your unbelief: for verily I say unto you, if ye have faith as a grain of mustard seed, ye shall say unto this mountain, Remove hence to yonder place; and it shall remove; and nothing shall be impossible unto you. ²¹ Howbeit this kind goeth not out but by prayer and fasting

Chapter 13: Fasting and Prayer

If you want to really get serious about prayer than there's no better way than to add fasting to your prayer life. Fasting and prayer can be found throughout both the Old Testament and the New Testament. Fasting and prayer are normally related to drawling close to God and seeking a breakthrough in a particular situation. Let's take a look at some examples of fasting and prayer in the Bible.

Ezra 8:21-22

[21] Then **I proclaimed a fast** there at the river of Ahava, **that we might humble ourselves before our God, to seek from Him the right way for us and our little ones and all our possessions.** [22] For I was ashamed to request of the king an escort of soldiers and horsemen to help us against the enemy on the road, because we had spoken to the king, saying, "The hand of our God *is* upon all those for good who seek Him, but His power and His wrath *are* against all those who forsake Him."

In Ezra we can see that the purpose of fasting and praying was to humble their cells before God and to seek God's direction for them and their families. I'm sure many of us can relate to wanting to know what the right path is.

We can see from Scripture that fasting and praying is a way for us to humble ourselves, lean not unto her own understanding, and seek God's direction for our lives. How many of us can truly say that we have done this? Draw close to God and he will draw close to you and you will know your path.

Psalms 35:11-14

> [11] Fierce witnesses rise up; They ask me *things* that I do not know. [12] They reward me evil for good, *To* the sorrow of my soul. [13] But as for me, when they were sick, My clothing *was* sackcloth; I humbled myself with fasting; And my prayer would return to my own heart. [14] I paced about as though *he were* my friend *or* brother; I bowed down heavily, as one who mourns *for his* mother.

In Psalms 35 we again see fasting as a way to humble ourselves before God Almighty. We can also see that prayer comes from the heart. The Scriptures declare, "Out of the abundance of the heart the mouth speaks" – (Matt. 12:34 / Luke 6:45) is a critical spiritual principle or law if you would – for in the power of the tongue there is life and there is death (Proverbs 18:21), speak life! Speak life to your situations, circumstances and call those things that are not as if they are according to the word of God – this is the essence of faith.

Now **faith is the** substance of things hoped for, **the evidence** of things not seen (Heb. 11:13)

[6] But without faith it is impossible to please him: for he that cometh to God must believe that he is, and that he is a rewarder of them that diligently seek him (Heb. 11:6).

[27] And Jesus looking upon them saith, With men it is impossible, but not with God: for with God all things are possible (Mark 10:27)

¹¹ Not that I speak in respect of want: for I have learned, in whatsoever state I am, therewith to be content. ¹² I know both how to be abased, and I know how to abound: every where and in all things I am instructed both to be full and to be hungry, both to abound and to suffer need. ¹³ I can do all things through Christ which strengtheneth me (Philippians 4:11-13)

Daniel 9:2-22

²In the first year of his reign I, Daniel, understood by the books the number of the years *specified* by the word of the Lord through Jeremiah the prophet, that He would accomplish seventy years in the desolations of Jerusalem.

³ Then I set my face toward the Lord God to make request by prayer and supplications, with fasting, sackcloth, and ashes. ⁴ And I prayed to the Lord my God, and made confession, and said, "O Lord, great and awesome God, who keeps His covenant and mercy with those who love Him, and with those who keep His commandments, ⁵ we have sinned and committed iniquity, we have done wickedly and rebelled, even by departing from Your precepts and Your judgments. ⁶ Neither have we heeded Your servants the prophets, who spoke in Your name to our kings and our princes, to our fathers and all the people of the land. ⁷ O Lord, righteousness *belongs* to You, but to us shame of face, as *it is* this day—to the men of Judah, to the inhabitants of Jerusalem and all Israel, those near and those far off in all the countries to which You have driven them, because of the unfaithfulness which they have committed against You. ⁸ "O Lord, to us *belongs* shame of face, to our kings, our princes, and our fathers, because we have sinned against You. ⁹To the Lord our God *belong* mercy and forgiveness, though we have rebelled against Him.

¹⁰ We have not obeyed the voice of the Lord our God, to walk in His laws, which He set before us by His servants the prophets. ¹¹ Yes, all Israel has transgressed Your law, and has departed so as not to obey Your voice; therefore the curse and the oath written in the Law of Moses the servant of God have been poured out on us, because we have sinned against Him.

¹² And He has confirmed His words, which He spoke against us and against our judges who judged us, by bringing upon us a great disaster; for under the whole heaven such has never been done as what has been done to Jerusalem. ¹³ "As *it is* written in the Law of Moses, all this disaster has come upon us; yet we have not made our prayer before the Lord our God, that we might turn from our iniquities and understand Your truth. ¹⁴Therefore the Lord has kept the disaster in mind, and brought it upon us; for the Lord our God *is* righteous in all the works which He does, though we have not obeyed His voice.

¹⁵And now, O Lord our God, who brought Your people out of the land of Egypt with a mighty hand, and made Yourself a name, as *it is* this day—we have sinned, we have done wickedly!

¹⁶ O Lord, according to all Your righteousness, I pray, let Your anger and Your fury be turned away from Your city Jerusalem, Your holy mountain; because for our sins, and for the iniquities of our fathers, Jerusalem and Your people *are* a reproach to all *those* around us. ¹⁷ Now therefore, our God, hear the prayer of Your servant, and his supplications, and for the Lord's sake cause Your face to shine on Your sanctuary, which is desolate. ¹⁸ O my God, incline Your ear and hear; open Your eyes and see our desolations, and the city which is called by Your name; for we do not present our supplications before You because of our righteous deeds, but because of Your great mercies.

¹⁹ O Lord, hear! O Lord, forgive! O Lord, listen and act! Do not delay for Your own sake, my God, for Your city and Your people are called by Your name." ²⁰ Now while I *was* speaking, praying, and confessing my sin and the sin of my people Israel, and presenting my supplication before the Lord my God for the holy mountain of my God, ²¹ yes, while I *was* speaking in prayer, the man Gabriel, whom I had seen in the vision at the beginning, being caused to fly swiftly, reached me about the time of the evening offering. ²² And he informed *me,* and talked with me, and said, "O Daniel, I have now come forth to give you skill to understand.

> The Scripture in Daniel 9 is a great example of how to pray for your country. Though God was talking specifically to Solomon regarding the house of the Lord we can see from Daniel chapter 9 that Daniel still prayed according to 2 Chon. 7:14. I'm sure a lot of you reading this book probably know the Scripture by heart but how many of us have fasted and prayed like Daniel to seek a healing for the land. Understand to heal the land requires that each of us are healed ourselves internally and spiritually.

¹⁴ If my people, which are called by my name, shall humble themselves, and pray, and seek my face, and turn from their wicked ways; then will I hear from heaven, and will forgive their sin, and will heal their land - (2 Chron. 7:14).

Matthew 17:20-21 Mark 9:28-29

²⁰ And Jesus said unto them, Because of your unbelief: for verily I say unto you, If ye have faith as a grain of mustard seed, ye shall say unto this mountain, Remove hence to yonder place; and it shall remove; and nothing shall be impossible unto you. ²¹ Howbeit this kind goeth not out but by prayer and fasting.

As we can see without faith you will have no victory in spiritual warfare. And remember, without faith it is impossible to please God – the One who enlisted you in His army. But make no mistake about it we will endure hardship as a good soldier of Jesus Christ according to Scripture –(2 Tim 2:3).However, hardship is not defeat it is just merely part of the war that were all in and some battles leave us more wounded than others. Nevertheless we have the victory in Christ regardless of how wounded we get.

Having the proper mindset is critical and this mindset comes from transforming yourself into the word of God, not the Word of God transforming itself into today's societal norms. Remember, heaven and earth will pass away but God's Word will remain the same – (Matt. 24:35).

It's important that we don't get discouraged in the battle, going back to the mindset once again.

Could you imagine the confusion of the apostles had when they attempted to invoke the name of Jesus and the demon wasn't cast out? Why did this happen? Jesus says this happen because of two things – their unbelief and the fact that this particular type of demon only comes out through fasting and prayer. I would speculate that because of the fierceness of this particular demon, because the apostles believe the lie of the physical world, of what they saw they were moved in their heart to believe that this demon is too strong. I believe this is the essence of where their unbelief stemmed from.

Now this is just speculation based off of reading the Scriptures no one can be entirely sure where of their unbelief stemmed from but it did originate from somewhere.

Additionally Jesus indicated that this particular type of demon only comes out through fasting and prayer. Now was He specifically talking regarding the apostles because of their unbelief or can this be universally applied? I tend to look at it like this – because of the apostles unbelief they needed to humble themselves before God by fasting and then pray for the demon to be removed. Because the Scriptures very clearly tell us that Christ has given us all authority over the enemy.

Let's review this real quick:

> Then He called His twelve disciples together and gave them power and authority over **all demons**, and to cure diseases. ² He sent them to preach the kingdom of God and to heal the sick - (Luke 9:1-2)

¹⁸ And He said to them, "I saw Satan fall like lightning from heaven. ¹⁹ Behold, I give you the authority to trample on serpents and scorpions, **and over all the power of the enemy**, and nothing shall by any means hurt you. ²⁰ Nevertheless do not rejoice in this, that the spirits are subject to you, but rather rejoice because your names are written in heaven." – (Luke 10:18-20).

The main thing to remember about the Scripture is to have faith, real faith and if you're struggling with faith pray and ask God to give you the faith that's needed to do his will each and every day. It's not just enough to know about God or to even read a book about God – you have to believe in your hearts and then confessed publicly with your mouth - (Rom 10:9-10).

Strongholds of the enemy may be present in your life or in a situation during which time is highly recommended if you want to have the victory over these things that you fast and pray.

Luke 2:36-38

> ³⁶ And there was one Anna, a prophetess, the daughter of Phanuel, of the tribe of Aser: she was of a great age, and had lived with an husband seven years from her virginity; ³⁷ And she was a widow of about fourscore and four years, which departed not from the temple, but served God with fastings and prayers night and day. ³⁸ And she coming in that instant gave thanks likewise unto the Lord, and spake of him to all them that looked for redemption in Jerusalem.

Here we see a combination of a virtuous woman and a prayer warrior. The Scriptures indicate that she was a woman of honor who followed the word of God even after her husband's death. We can see her dedication to the Lord in the fact that she did not depart from the temple but served God with fastings and prayers both day and night all the meanwhile continuingly telling people where they can find redemption – a powerful woman of God.

Luke 5:33-35

³³ And they said unto him, Why do the disciples of John fast often, and make prayers, and likewise the disciples of the Pharisees; but thine eat and drink? ³⁴ And he said unto them, Can ye make the children of the bride chamber fast, while the bridegroom is with them? **³⁵ But the days will come, when the bridegroom shall be taken away from them, and then shall they fast in those days.**

> Brothers and sisters we are in the days Jesus spoke about, the days in which we shall fast and pray. When is the last time you fasted and prayed? If you're truly serious about being a prayer warrior, if you want to take your prayer life to the next level, if you want to draw close to God than it's time to start fasting and praying on a more regular basis.

Now obviously if you have specific medical needs or conditions it's important to consult with your primary doctor to ensure that it is safe for you to fast. If you do have medical conditions that preclude you from completely fasting then maybe consider a juice fast. A juice fast requires the use of a juicer that processes vegetables and fruits into pure juice without the pulp and the fiber.

This is a great way to get started with fasting because not only are you fasting from particular items that you would normally eat but you're also doing something that will promote the overall health and well-being of your body – the temple of the living God.

1 Cor 7:2-5

2 Nevertheless, to avoid fornication, let every man have his own wife, and let every woman have her own husband. 3 Let the husband render unto the wife due benevolence: and likewise also the wife unto the husband.

4 The wife hath not power of her own body, but the husband: and likewise also the husband hath not power of his own body, but the wife. **5 Defraud ye not one the other, except it be with consent for a time, that ye may give yourselves to fasting and prayer;** and come together again, that Satan tempt you not for your incontinency.

The above Scripture is very interesting when we understand that the two become one in the flesh (Matt.19:5 / Mark 10:8 / 1 Cor. 6:16 / Eph. 5:31). However, the fact that the two become one in the flesh does not mean they come together as one in the spirit.

Though the two are one in the flesh it is clear that each one has to work out our own salvation with fear and trembling before the Lord – (Philippians 2:12)

Scripture indicates not to withhold the love that is due one another except with consent for a time that you may give yourself to fasting and prayer and then come together again. There are some key points that we should address here:

First and foremost there needs to be permission given – an agreement prior to restraining from giving yourself to one another.

Secondly there is a time that is indicated in the agreement whether it's a day a week, whatever it is it is verbally articulated and agreed to by both parties.

The only time this is permitted is for fasting and prayer

You must come together immediately following your fast and prayer to ensure you are not tempted.

Chapter 14: Prayer - Conclusion

It's up to each one of us to actively get into the fight, or maybe more importantly realize there is a war going on spiritually and we are all in a battle for our very souls. For the scriptures declare to "Wherefore, my beloved, as ye have always obeyed, not as in my presence only, but now much more in my absence, work out your own salvation with fear and trembling - Philippians 2:12"

This is a real war in the Spiritual realm that continues to bleed over into the physical world. So many men and women of God aren't even in the fight because they refuse to address their sin and run to God for forgiveness, let me tell you now – "As long as there is breath in Your lungs there is Hope in God for Change" – AJF

We must all do what we can, when we can, as God enables us

From personally getting right with God, to effectively leading, guiding and protecting your family, to even effecting your community, society, and ultimately the world. Christians have forgotten what the "Far Left" has not – That one person can make a difference in the world and united we become stronger.

Why have Christians forgotten this critical lesson from History

– Do we not remember that 12 men (Christ and the 11 Apostles – I don't really count Judas) Changed the World. We as Christian need to walk in that same boldness that they have walked in, that same Spirit of Conviction, Compassion, and Love. There is a time for everything under heaven and as you draw close to Jesus Christ the Holy Spirit will continually lead and guide you. The Question is do you really have Faith –

If you really have Faith you will "Take Action for the Kingdom of God". I challenge you to examine if you are in fact in the faith and to walk courageously, yes boldly in the Word of God for His name's sake. If we want to all make America great again then it's going to have to start with a transformation of each of our hearts and the hearts of those that claim to follow Christ – and that starts with Prayer.

What does the Scriptures say, "If my people, which are called by my name, shall **humble themselves, and Pray**, and seek my face, and turn from their wicked ways; then will I hear from heaven, and will forgive their sin, and will heal their land. 2 Chronicles 7:14"

The time is now – "Take Action for the Kingdom of God" and get about the Father's business for tomorrow is never promised.

"Think For Yourself and Learn Directly From God"

If you've learned nothing else in reading this book you've learned that without prayer our spiritual lives are basically non- existent. We cannot know God if we do not speak to Him and listen to Him. We cannot speak or listen to Him if we do not pray. There is a major difference between knowing God and being known by God.

Before I end this I also want to leave you with this scriptural truth: God hears and answers each and every prayer we say. Silent or out loud. Big or small concerns. He hears and answers them all. His answers may not always be what we want, but they will always be what we need

God bless each and every one of you who have read this book - know that I pray for all You as my Brother or Sister in Christ and that you are Not Alone in the War and together we can make a difference.

Special Gift

God has a Gift for You!   The Plan of Salvation:

There is no formal prayer of salvation as many churches would have you believe, God's Word is very clear - there is only one way to get to the Father in heaven and that is through Jesus Christ (John 14:6). Jesus says that you must be born again to enter into heaven (John 3:3-5).

Salvation is simply the first step in building an open and honest relationship with God. We all have sinned and fallen short, but there is Hope in Jesus Christ - Just cry out to God in sincerity and honesty asking for forgiveness and for Him to Save you, Sanctify you, and fill you with His Holy Spirit - Ask for His will to be done in your life on earth as it is in Heaven and That's it, now just keep it real with God.

A Warning:

The Christian walk is not an easy life on the surface. The Word of God says that we will be hated in all the world for Christ namesake (Matt. 24:9). The Bible says that in the last days are enemy prevail against us physically until Christ returns to save us (Dan 7:21, 22). Furthermore, we must endure hardship as a good soldier of Jesus Christ (2 Tim 2:3) and yet we are never alone in this, God promises us that He will never leave us nor forsake us if we believe in him (Matt.28:20).

In everything we go through we have the peace and joy of God which surpasses all understanding (Philp. 4:6-8) The Bible declares, "For I consider the sufferings of this present time are not worthy to be compared with the glory which shall be revealed in us". (Rom 8:18). However, in all these things we are more than conquerors through Jesus Christ (Rom. 8:37)

Stay in Contact

Stay in Contact with the American Christian Defense Alliance, Inc. through Our Website At: ACDAInc.Org

Join Our Mailing List

We also Greatly Appreciate You Signing Up For Our Mailing List and Providing a Good Rating and review for this Book. Your reviews help other people like yourself find this book and benefit from its contents.

If You or Your Family have been Blessed by this book please let us know by dropping us a line through our website at ACDAInc.Org

Find All Our Books

Some of Our Books:

Parenting: How To Be A Great Parent And Raise Awesome Kids

Prayer: Your No. 1 Prayer Book To Learn To Be A Strong Christian Prayer Warrior That Prays With Powerful Prayers In The War Room To Overcome And Defeat The Enemy

Salvation for Your Unsaved Mom: 10 Things to Tell Your Mom Before She Dies

Wisdom from Your Elders: Learning From Your Parents, Grandparents, and the Older People in Your Church

Kids and Prayer: Pray with Your Kids and Teach Them How to Pray

Embrace Your Special Needs Child, Prayer, and Parenting

Embracing Pregnancy, Your Child, and Parenting: A Christian Parenting Guide to Offer Encouragement During the Wonders, Joy, and Hope of Your First Child

Race Relations in America: A Christian Guide to Unite Christians in the Faith

Martial Arts Ministry: How To Start A Martial Arts Ministry

Biblical Bug Out: Don't Bug In - Follow The Calling

Christian Prepping 101: How To Start Prepping

How to Finance Your Full-Time RV Dream

Make Money: A Beginners Guide to Start an Online Business, Work from Home, Make Money, and Develop Financial Freedom

Additional Formats

Thank you for reading this book. Your support and the support of others continue to humble us and enable our Ministry to grow. We hope and pray that this book has blessed you in some way. If you enjoyed this book consider purchasing it as a gift for someone who could benefit from it.

We Greatly Appreciate Your Support as Well as You Sharing this information, including links to our books with Others on Your Social Media Platforms

Thank You Once Again for Your Support; We Know God Will Bless You as You Have Blessed This Ministry

www.ingramcontent.com/pod-product-compliance
Lightning Source LLC
Chambersburg PA
CBHW021351210526
45463CB00001B/65